EVALUATING FEDERAL RESEARCH PROGRAMS

Research and the Government Performance and Results Act

Committee on Science, Engineering, and Public Policy

National Academy of Sciences
National Academy of Engineering
Institute of Medicine

NATIONAL ACADEMY PRESS
Washington, D.C. 1999

NATIONAL ACADEMY PRESS • 2101 Constitution Ave., NW • Washington, DC 20418

NOTICE: This volume was produced as part of a project approved by the Governing Board of the National Research Council, whose members are drawn from the councils of the National Academy of Sciences, the National Academy of Engineering, and the Institute of Medicine. It is a result of work done by the Committee on Science, Engineering, and Public Policy (COSEPUP) as augmented, which has authorized its release to the public. This report has been reviewed by a group other than the authors according to procedures approved by COSEPUP and the Report Review Committee.

The National Academy of Sciences (NAS) is a private, nonprofit, self-perpetuating society of distinguished scholars engaged in scientific and engineering research, dedicated to the furtherance of science and technology and to their use for the general welfare. Under the authority of the charter granted to it by Congress in 1863, the Academy has a working mandate that calls on it to advise the federal government on scientific and technical matters. Dr. Bruce M. Alberts is president of NAS.

The National Academy of Engineering (NAE) was established in 1964, under the charter of NAS, as a parallel organization of distinguished engineers. It is autonomous in its administration and in the selection of members, sharing with NAS its responsibilities for advising the federal government. The National Academy of Engineering also sponsors engineering programs aimed at meeting national needs, encourages education and research, and recognizes the superior achievements of engineers. Dr. William A. Wulf is president of NAE.

The Institute of Medicine (IOM) was established in 1970 by NAS to secure the services of eminent members of appropriate professions in the examination of policy matters pertaining to the health of the public. The Institute acts under the responsibility given to NAS in its congressional charter to be an adviser to the federal government and, on its own initiative, to identify issues of medical care, research, and education. Dr. Kenneth I. Shine is president of IOM.

The Committee on Science, Engineering, and Public Policy (COSEPUP) is a joint committee of NAS, NAE, and IOM. It includes members of the councils of all three bodies.

Financial Support: The development of this report was supported by the National Research Council, the National Science Foundation, the National Institutes of Health, the National Aeronautics and Space Administration, the Department of Agriculture, the Department of Transportation, and the Department of Defense.

International Standard Book Number 0-309-06430-9

Limited copies are available from: Committee on Science, Engineering, and Public Policy, 2101 Constitution Ave., NW, Washington, DC 20418.

Additional copies are available for sale from: National Academy Press, Box 285, 2101 Constitution Ave., NW, Washington, DC 20055. You may order by phone at 1-800-624-6242 (202-334-3313 in the Washington metropolitan area) or by visiting the National Academy Press web site, www.nap.edu.

Printed in the United States of America

COMMITTEE ON SCIENCE, ENGINEERING, AND PUBLIC POLICY

PHILLIP A. GRIFFITHS,* (Chair), Director, Institute for Advanced Study, Princeton, New Jersey
BRUCE M. ALBERTS,* President, National Academy of Sciences, Washington, D.C.
PETER DIAMOND, Professor of Economics, Massachusetts Institute of Technology, Cambridge
GERALD DINNEEN,* Retired Vice President, Science and Technology, Honeywell, Inc., Edina, Minnesota
MILDRED S. DRESSELHAUS, Institute Professor of Electrical Engineering and Physics, Massachusetts Institute of Technology, Cambridge
JAMES J. DUDERSTADT, President Emeritus and University Professor of Science and Engineering, Millennium Project, University of Michigan, Ann Arbor
MARYE ANNE FOX, Chancellor, North Carolina State University, Raleigh
RALPH E. GOMORY, President, Alfred P. Sloan Foundation, New York, New York
RUBY P. HEARN, Vice President, The Robert Wood Johnson Foundation, Princeton, New Jersey
PHILIP W. MAJERUS, Professor of Medicine, Biochemistry, and Molecular Biophysics and Director, Division of Hematology-Oncology, Washington University School of Medicine, St. Louis, Missouri
JUNE E. OSBORN, President, Josiah Macy, Jr. Foundation, New York, New York
KENNETH I. SHINE,* President, Institute of Medicine, Washington, D.C.
MORRIS TANENBAUM, Retired Vice Chairman and Chief Financial Officer, AT&T, Short Hills, New Jersey
WILLIAM JULIUS WILSON, Malcolm Wiener Professor, Center for Social Policy, John F. Kennedy School of Government, Harvard University, Cambridge, Massachusetts
WILLIAM A. WULF,* President, National Academy of Engineering, Washington, D.C.

*Ex officio member

RICHARD BISSELL, Executive Director
DEBORAH D. STINE, Associate Director and Study Director
ANNE-MARIE MAZZA, Senior Program Officer
BRETT WILLETTE, Research Associate
CAROLYN RYAN, Research Associate
MARION RAMSEY, Administrative Associate
SUSAN COZZENS, Consultant
ALAN ANDERSON, Consultant Science Writer
NORMAN GROSSBLATT, Editor

PREFACE

The 1993 Government Performance and Results Act ("the Results Act," or GPRA) requires federal agencies to set strategic goals and to use performance measures for management and budgeting. The objective of GPRA is to encourage greater efficiency, effectiveness, and accountability in federal programs and spending. Development of plans to implement the act has been particularly difficult for agencies responsible for research activities supported by the federal government because of the difficulty of linking results with annual investments in research. The Committee on Science, Engineering, and Public Policy (COSEPUP) of the National Academy of Sciences, the National Academy of Engineering, and the Institute of Medicine is conducting a three-part study to:

1. Identify and analyze the most effective ways to assess the results of research, on the basis of consultation with federal agencies, oversight entities, the research community, industry, states, and agencies of other nations.
2. Help the federal government determine how its agencies can better incorporate research activities in strategic and performance plans and improve the management and effectiveness of research programs, including a determination of what can be reliably measured and the best mechanism for doing so, a determination of what cannot be measured, an evaluation of the extent to which common analytic paradigms could be used across agencies for assessing the results of extramural and intramural research programs and of the training and education of the scientific and engineering

workforce, development of such paradigms if feasible, and development of implementation principles and guidelines that could assist Congress and the Office of Management and Budget (OMB) in reviewing agency performance plans.

3. Develop mechanisms to evaluate the effects of implementing GPRA on agency program decisions and on the practices of research, which requires COSEPUP to identify lessons learned and best practices that could be used by other agencies or programs and to determine effective ways for Congress and OMB to use the results of these plans. The committee plans to begin its work on the third charge in the Spring of 1999.

The current study, which addresses parts 1 and 2 described above, began in January 1998. During Part 1 of the study, COSEPUP held three workshops: the first focused on industry methods to evaluate the performance of research, the second on agencies' strategic and performance plans, and the third on methods to evaluate the outcomes of research. Each workshop provided valuable information and a chance for input from all interested parties, including the agencies, the Office of Science and Technology Policy, OMB, congressional committees, the General Accounting Office, disciplinary societies, and researchers. The committee thanks all those who attended for their valuable participation.

The first workshop indicated that applied research is pursued widely in technology-based industries, is focused on achieving well-defined practical outcomes, and is planned and measured in ways similar to ways that other high-risk business undertakings are planned and measured—with business cases, risk-adjusted rate-of-return requirements, and so on. Basic research, where it is still supported by industry, is focused on well-defined areas when such work is judged to be able to lead to technological breakthroughs. Basic research programs also serve as a human resource pool for a firm and as a working contact with similar basic research performed worldwide. Basic research is supported and evaluated on the basis of how well it serves those purposes, that is, is the work relevant to the firm's future? Is it of high quality? Are the best people recruited to do it?

The second workshop demonstrated the wide range of procedures and methods that agencies have used in responding to GPRA's requirements for planning programs and measuring outcomes. Because applied research programs by definition have desired outcomes directly related to agency missions, evaluating such programs can be relatively straightforward and agencies can use methods similar to those used by industry. We found variations of these methods in place in some agencies and recommend that they be fully and consistently used. It became clear, however, that substantial problems existed for agencies trying to evaluate basic research programs. Urgent concern was expressed that basic research could not be effectively evaluated in the context of GPRA and that misguided attempts to do so could cause great damage. We strongly agree that misguided attempts must be avoided, and we recommend how evaluation can be meaningfully performed.

Since measuring the outcomes from basic research is the most troublesome for the agencies and, in COSEPUP's opinion, the most crucial issue for the long-term economic health of the nation, it has received the most attention in this report. We also deal with measuring the outcomes of applied research and the question of the coordination of planning for all federal research programs.

COSEPUP received encouragement in conducting this study from Representatives F. James Sensenbrenner, Jr., (chair, House Science Committee) and George Brown (member and former chair of the House Science Committee). In a letter (Appendix B) from them, they described the broad range of issues that they see for the planning and evaluation of research in the context of GPRA. This study addresses a portion of those issues, and future work will address other portions.

We have limited this discussion to general principles. Each of our recommendations requires specific guidelines for implementation, and we have not attempted to provide such guidelines in this report. Because GPRA is in operation today with annual reporting and planning requirements, it seemed important to state general principles as soon as possible and, to the degree that they are acceptable, to direct future work to provide more specific recommendations on implementation. Following the release of this report, COSEPUP will arrange meetings and workshops with agency representatives, congressional staff, and oversight bodies to identify the recommendations they would like COSEPUP to develop further.

PHILLIP A. GRIFFITHS
Chair
Committee on Science, Engineering, and Public Policy

ACKNOWLEDGMENTS

This report has benefited from input from various individuals. COSEPUP acknowledges those who made presentations at the workshops and panel discussions: John McTague, Ford Motor Company; Pradip Das, Analytical Sciences Center, Monsanto; Melvin Cohen, Lucent Technologies; David Thomas, Amoco Corporation; Rajen Dalal, Chiron Corporation; Charles Larson, Industrial Research Institute, Inc.; David Rust, George Cooper, Tom Sexton, Bob MacDonald, and Sally Rockey, U.S. Department of Agriculture; Ernest Moniz, Patricia Dehmer, and Robert Astheimer, U.S. Department of Energy; Harold Varmus, Lana Skirboll, John Uzzell, and Wendy Baldwin, National Institutes of Health; Alan Ladwig and Gary Steinberg, National Aeronautics and Space Administration; Neal Lane, Judy Sunley, and Dave Schindel, National Science Foundation; Bob Trew, Joanna Spriggs, and Ed Brown, U.S. Department of Defense; Dani Brzezinska, Fenton Carey, and Paula Ewen, U.S. Department of Transportation; Kevin Teichman, Environmental Protection Agency; Curt Marshall, National Oceanic and Atmospheric Administration; William Ott and Paul Doremus, National Institute of Standards and Technology; T.J. Glauthier and Sarah Horrigan, Office of Management and Budget; Beverly Hartline, Office of Science and Technology Policy; Phillip Kiko, Beth Sokul, and Scott Rayder, House Science Committee; Robert Simon, Senator Jeff Bingaman's office; Genevieve Knezo, Congressional Research Service; Susan Kladiva, General Accounting Office; Henry Small, Institute for Scientific Information; Al Link, University of North Carolina; Irwin Feller, Pennsylvania State University; Paul David, Stanford University and Oxford; Barry Bozeman, Georgia Institute of Technology; and Deborah Boehm-Davis, George Mason University. In addition, COSEPUP would like to thank all those who attended the workshops for their valuable participation

This report has been reviewed by persons chosen for their diverse perspectives and technical expertise in accordance with procedures approved by the National Research Council's Report Review Committee. The purposes of this independent review are to provide candid and critical comments that will assist COSEPUP in making its report as sound as possible and to ensure that the report meets institutional standards of objectivity, evidence, and responsiveness to the study charge. The review comments and draft manuscript remain confidential to protect the integrity of the deliberative process. We wish to thank the following for their participation in the review of this report:

Harvey Bernstein, Barry Bozeman, Rad Byerly, Linda Capuano, Irwin Feller, William Gordon, Paul Gray, Marcelle LaFollette, Stephen Lukasik, Bill Morrill, Ann Peterson, Robert Shannon, Christine Sloane, Bob White, and the report review coordinator, Anita Jones.

Although those persons have provided many constructive comments and suggestions, responsibility for the final content of this report rests solely with COSEPUP.

The production of the report was the result of hard work by the committee as a whole and by the extra effort of the Guidance Group consisting of Peter Diamond, Gerald Dinneen, Mildred Dresselhaus, Ralph Gomory, Philip Majerus, Kenneth Shine, Morris Tanenbaum, and me, co chaired by Ralph Gomory and Morris Tanenbaum, which convened between regular COSEPUP meetings.

The project was aided by the invaluable help of COSEPUP professional staff—Deborah D. Stine, associate director of COSEPUP; Anne-Marie Mazza, senior program officer; Brett Willette, research associate; Carolyn Ryan, research associate;

Michael Hostetler, intern, and its consultants, Susan Cozzens, who provided guidance to the committee on GPRA, and Alan Anderson, science writer. They all helped to draft and revise the report throughout the project. The committee also thanks Richard Bissell, executive director of COSEPUP, who oversaw the committee's activities, and the report's diligent editor, Norman Grossblatt.

PHILLIP A. GRIFFITHS
Chair
Committee on Science, Engineering, and Public Policy

CONTENTS

EXECUTIVE SUMMARY

The Government Performance and Results Act (GPRA), enacted in 1993, focuses agency and oversight attention on the performance and results of government activities by requiring that all federal agencies measure and report on the results of their activities annually. Agencies are required to develop a strategic plan that sets goals and objectives for at least a 5-year period, an annual performance plan that translates the goals of the strategic plan into annual targets, and an annual performance report that demonstrates whether the targets are met. The Committee on Science, Engineering, and Public Policy (COSEPUP) of the National Academy of Sciences, the National Academy of Engineering, and the Institute of Medicine has addressed the issue of measuring and evaluating research in compliance with the requirements of GPRA.

COSEPUP recognizes the opportunities and challenges that GPRA presents for agencies that invest in research. GPRA offers those agencies the opportunity to communicate to policymakers and the public the rationale for and results of their research programs. At the same time, GPRA presents substantial challenges to the agencies.

During the course of this study, COSEPUP held several workshops. In these workshops and in other input to the committee, we have heard two distinct and conflicting viewpoints on approaches to measuring basic research. One is that it should be possible to measure research, including basic research, annually and provide quantitative measures of the useful outcomes of both basic and applied research. The other is that, given the long-range nature of basic research, there is no sensible way to respond to the GPRA annual measurement requirement and that the best that can be done is to provide measures that appear to respond but in fact are essentially meaningless, such as a list of an agency's top 100 discoveries of the preceding year.

COSEPUP's view, spelled out in more detail in what follows, is different from both those viewpoints. In essence, our report takes two strong positions. First, the useful outcomes of basic research cannot be measured directly on an annual basis, because the usefulness of new basic knowledge is inherently too unpredictable; so the usefulness of basic research must be measured by historical reviews based on a much longer timeframe. Second, that does not mean that there are no meaningful measures of performance of basic research while the research is in progress; in fact, the committee believes that there are meaningful measures of quality, relevance, and leadership that are good predictors of eventual usefulness, that these measures can be reported regularly, and that they represent a sound way to ensure that the country is getting a good return on its basic research investment.

The problem of reporting on applied research is much simpler: it consists of systematically applying methods widely used in industry and in some parts of government. For example, an applied research program usually includes a series of milestones that should be achieved by particular times and a description of the intended final outcomes and their significance. Periodic reporting can indicate progress toward those milestones.

The remainder of this executive summary provides a more in-depth description of COSEPUP's conclusions and recommendations regarding how to evaluate federal research programs relative to GPRA. It also addresses coordination among federal research programs and human-resource issues. COSEPUP concludes that both basic research and applied research programs[1] can be meaningfully evaluated on a regular basis. For the applied research programs of the mission agencies, specific practical outcomes can be documented and progress toward their achievement can be measured annually. For example, if the Department of Energy adopted the goal of producing cheaper solar energy, it could measure the results of research directed toward decreasing the cost of solar cells; this applied research project would be evaluated annually against specific measurable milestones. However, the practical outcomes of basic research in science and engineering can seldom be identified while the research is in progress. Basic research has annual results that can be meaningfully evaluated, but these evaluations often do not give even a hint of ultimate practical outcomes.

History tells us unmistakably that by any measure, the benefit to the United States for leadership in basic research is extremely high—lives saved, inventions fostered, and jobs and wealth created. History also shows us how often basic research in science and engineering leads to outcomes that were unexpected or took many years or even decades to emerge. COSEPUP strongly believes that measures of the practical outcomes of basic research usually must be retrospective and historical and that the unpredictable nature of practical outcomes is an inherent and unalterable feature of basic research. For example, pre-World War II basic research on atomic structure contributed to today's Global Positioning System, an outcome of great practical and economic value, but, attempts to evaluate a year's worth of that early research even if they demonstrated high quality and world leadership, would have contained no hint of this particular outcome.

Since we cannot predict the ultimate practical outcomes of basic research, we must find ways to ensure that the basic research programs that the nation funds generate the kinds of knowledge that have given us great practical benefits in the past. To do that, we must find ways to measure the quality of our current research programs, their contributions to our world leadership in the relevant fields, and their relevance to agency goals and intended users.

World leadership is an important measure. In an earlier report (COSEPUP, 1993), COSEPUP recommended that, for the sake of the nation's well-being, the United States be among the leaders in all major fields of science and pre-eminent in selected fields of national importance. That is because a nation must be performing research at the forefront of a field if it is to understand, appropriate, and capitalize on current advances in that field, no matter where in the world they occur. New knowledge has value to nations where highly educated people performing cutting-edge research in the field of discovery can make use of the new knowledge when practical outcomes appear possible.

The people best qualified to evaluate basic or applied research are those with the knowledge and experience to understand its quality, and, in the case of applied research, its connection to public and agency goals. Evaluating basic research requires substantial scientific or engineering knowledge. Evaluating applied research requires, in addition, the ability to recognize its potential applicability to practical problems.

With those considerations in mind, COSEPUP has reached six conclusions and offers six recommendations regarding the evaluation of federally supported research programs.

Conclusion 1: Both applied research and basic research programs supported by the federal government can be evaluated meaningfully on a regular basis.

Conclusion 2: Agencies must evaluate their research programs by using measurements that match the character of the research. Differences in the character of the research will lead to differences in the appropriate timescale for measurement, in what is measurable and what is not, and in the expertise needed by those who contribute to the measurement process.

For applied research programs, progress toward specified practical outcomes can usually be measured annually by using milestones and other fairly standard approaches common in industry and in some parts of the federal government. For basic research, in contrast, progress toward practical outcomes cannot be measured annually, and attempts to measure such progress annually can in fact be harmful. Basic research progress can be reported annually in terms of quality, leadership, and relevance to agency goals, but practical outcomes can be measured only against a far longer historical perspective. In practical terms, because quality, leadership, and relevance will usually change slowly, the GPRA annual-reporting requirement can usually be met by minor updating of full evaluations that are done in a more flexible timeframe. There is a much greater chance that important events will take place in subfields, because of either scientific events or funding changes, so subprogram changes should constitute much of the updating.

Different expertise is required for measuring the worth of applied research and the worth of basic research. Measuring both requires technical and scientific knowledge, but applied research entails some factors that basic research does not, such as ultimate usability, so the input of potential users is required. That leads to our next conclusion.

Conclusion 3: The most effective means of evaluating federally funded research programs is expert review. Expert review—which includes quality review, relevance review, and benchmarking—should be used to assess both basic research and applied research programs.

Expert review is widely applied—used, for example, by congressional committees, by other professions, by industry boards, and throughout the realm of science and engineering—to answer complex questions through consultation with expert advisers. It is useful in helping an agency answer three kinds of questions of particular relevance to GPRA:

- What is the quality of the research program—for example, how good is current research work compared with other work being conducted in the field?[2] This question is best answered by reviewers who are sufficiently expert in the field being assessed to perform a *quality review*. This approach is traditionally called peer review. Peer review is commonly applied to projects, but here we are applying it to programs. The talent, objective judgment, and experience of these experts, or peers, are paramount and should be the criteria for their selection.
- Is the research program focused on the subjects most relevant to the agency mission? Another form of expert review is *relevance review*, in which potential users, joined by experts in related fields, evaluate the relevance of research to agency goals—is the research on subjects in which new understanding could be important in fulfilling the agency's mission? In reviewing the relevance of a program, a panel would assess the appropriateness of the direction of the research to the agency mission and its potential value to intended users.
- Is the research being performed at the forefront of scientific and technological knowledge? This is a relevant question for many programs, but it is particularly important for whole fields and subfields being supported. Evaluations of fields and subfields is best done through *international benchmarking* by a panel of experts who have sufficient stature and perspective to assess the international standing of research.

For agencies whose missions include a specific responsibility for basic research—such as the National Science Foundation in broad fields of science and engineering, the National Institutes of Health in fields related to health, or the Department of Energy in high-energy physics—world leadership in a field can itself be an agency goal. That is equally true for mission agencies, such as Department of Defense (DOD) but in more focused ways. For example, DOD can take as a goal world leadership in basic materials research relevant to its mission. Once such a goal is established, the usual measures of quality and leadership should be applied.

Conclusion 4: The nation cannot benefit from advances in science and technology without a continuing supply of well-educated and well-trained scientists and engineers. Without such a flow, the capability of an agency to fulfill its mission will be compromised. Agencies must pay increased attention to their human-resource requirements in terms of training and educating young scientists and engineers and in terms of providing an adequate supply of scientists and engineers to academe, industry, and federal laboratories.

Federal agencies that support research and exploit its results are able to do so because the education and training programs of the universities, in the course of performing much of that research, and the federal laboratories provide a continuing flow of qualified scientists and engineers. Even though section 1115(a)(3) of GPRA requires agencies to describe the human resources required to meet their performance goals, few agencies describe the importance of human resources or propose ways to ensure their adequacy in their strategic or performance plans.

Conclusion 5: Mechanisms for coordinating research programs in multiple agencies whose fields or subject matters overlap are insufficient.

It is common and valuable for agencies to approach similar fields of research from different perspectives. Indeed, this pluralism is a major strength of the U.S. research enterprise. But, better communication among agencies would enhance opportunities for collaboration, help keep important questions from being overlooked, and reduce instances of inefficient duplication of effort. Present mechanisms need strengthening.

Conclusion 6: The development of effective methods for evaluating and reporting performance requires the participation of the scientific and engineering community, whose members will necessarily be involved in expert review.

The researchers who work in agency, university, and industrial laboratories are the people who perform and best understand the research programs funded by the federal government. Many researchers contribute substantial time and effort to reviewing papers submitted for publication, grant applications, and program proposals, yet few of them are aware of GPRA, its objectives, and its mandates. Increased contact with and advice from the broader scientific and engineering community regarding the methods of determining and reporting quality and regarding the leadership position of agency research programs and the relevance of research to agency missions can benefit the GPRA process.

On the basis of those conclusions, COSEPUP offers the following recommendations:

Recommendation 1: Because both applied research and basic research can be evaluated meaningfully on a regular basis and are vital to research and mission agencies, research programs should be described in strategic and performance plans and evaluated in performance reports.

The performance of research is critical to the missions of many federal agencies. Therefore, a full description of an agency's goals and results, which is a principal objective of GPRA, must contain an evaluation of research activities and their relevance to the agency's mission.

Recommendation 2: For applied research programs, agencies should measure progress toward practical outcomes. For basic research programs, agencies should measure quality, relevance, and leadership. In addition, agencies should conduct periodic reviews of the overall practical outcomes of an agency's overall past support of applied and basic research. The use of measurements needs to recognize what can and cannot be measured. Misuse of measurement can lead to strongly negative results; for example, measuring basic research on the basis of short-term relevance would be extremely destructive to quality work.

Because the evaluation of applied research is directly connected to practical outcomes, whereas the evaluation of basic research is in terms of quality, relevance, and leadership, which ultimately lead to practical outcomes, there might be a tendency to bias an agency's overall research program toward applied research at the expense of basic research. This should be avoided, and a proper balance should be maintained.

Recommendation 3: Federal agencies should use expert review to assess the quality of research they support, the relevance of that research to their mission, and the leadership of the research. Expert review must strive for balance between having the most knowledgeable and the most independent individuals serve as members. Each agency should develop clear, explicit guidance with regard to structuring and employing expert review processes.

The most effective way to evaluate research programs is by expert review. The most commonly used form of expert review of quality is peer review. This operates on the premise that the people best qualified to judge the quality of research are experts in the field of research. This premise prevails across the research spectrum, from basic research to applied research. A second form of expert review is relevance review, in which potential users and experts in other fields or disciplines related to an agency's mission or to the potential application of the research evaluate the relevance of research to the agency's mission. A third form of expert review is benchmarking, in which an international panel of experts compares the level of leadership of a research program relative to research being performed worldwide.

Recommendation 4: Both research and mission agencies should describe in their strategic and performance plans the goal of developing and maintaining adequate human resources in fields critical to their missions both at the national level and in their agencies. Human resources should become a part of the evaluation of a research program along with the program's quality in terms of research advancement, relevance in terms of application development, and leadership in terms of the ability to take advantage of opportunities when they arise.

In early drafts of strategic and performance plans, agencies have generally omitted discussions of education and training, which are fundamental to the ability of agencies to fulfill their missions. The goal of developing and maintaining adequate human resources in fields critical to their missions should be supported by plans that produce that outcome. The nation cannot benefit from advances in science and technology without a continuing supply of well-educated and well-trained scientists and engineers. In addition, in the absence of such a flow, the capability of an agency to fulfill its mission will be compromised and the knowledge learned and technology developed will be lost.

Recommendation 5: Although GPRA is conducted agency-by-agency, a formal process should be established to identify and coordinate areas of research that are supported by multiple agencies. A lead agency should be identified for each field of research and that agency should be responsible for assuring that coordination occurs among the agencies.

It is common and valuable for multiple agencies to approach similar fields of research from different perspectives. Indeed, this pluralism is a major strength of the U.S. research enterprise. However, better communication among agencies would enhance opportunities for collaboration, help to keep important questions from being overlooked, and reduce instances of inefficient duplication of effort. A single agency should be identified to serve as the focal point for each particular field of research so that all significant supported fields are covered. Information regarding support for that field should be provided to all the agencies involved in it so that they can adjust their efforts to ensure that the field is appropriately covered. Agencies should use benchmarking, which affords the opportunity to look across fields, in their efforts to understand the status of a particular field of research.

Recommendation 6: The science and engineering community can and should play an important role in GPRA implementation. As a first step, they should become familiar with agency strategic and performance plans, which are available on the agencies' web sites.

The researchers who work in agency, university, and industrial laboratories are the people who perform and best understand the research programs funded by the federal government. Many researchers contribute substantial time and effort to reviewing papers submitted for publication, grant applications, and program proposals, but few of them are aware of GPRA. Their greater involvement in implementing GPRA would be beneficial to the country. Increased contact with and advice from the broader scientific and engineering community regarding both the quality and the leadership position of agency research programs and the relevance of the research to agency missions can benefit the GPRA process.

COSEPUP intends to address mechanisms and guidelines for implementing these recommendations in workshops and meetings with representatives from federal agencies, Congress, OMB, and oversight bodies. Given the diverse portfolio of research conducted by federal agencies and the urgency of addressing the question of how basic research can be evaluated in the context of GPRA, the level of detail and specificity needed in designing procedures and guidelines for implementation was beyond the scope of this report.

The Government Performance and Results Act provides an opportunity for the research community to ensure the effective use of the nation's research resources in meeting national needs and to articulate to policy-makers and the public the rationale for and results of research. We believe that our recommendations can assist federal agencies in complying with GPRA.

NOTES

1. For purposes of this study, *program* refers to a set of activities focused on a particular area that can include multiple projects with different risks, time horizons, and outcomes.

2. There are at least two aspects of quality—one absolute and one relative. The absolute aspects are related to the quality of the research plan, the methods by which it is being pursued, its role in education when conducted at a university, and the importance of its results to its sponsor, either obtained or expected. The relative aspects pertain to its leadership at the edge of an advancing field. Although the leadership aspect is generally important, the results might in some cases be of great importance to an agency albeit not at the leading edge of a field.

CHAPTER 1

STATEMENT OF THE PROBLEM

GPRA and Research

In 1993, Congress passed the Government Performance and Results Act (GPRA) with broad bipartisan support. The law is part of a set of budget-reform measures intended to increase the effectiveness and efficiency of government. Both the General Accounting Office (GAO) and the Office of Management and Budget (OMB) testified in favor of the bill, and the President's National Performance Review advocated its implementation. Unlike several predecessor systems (program planning and budgeting, management by objectives, and zero-based budgeting), GPRA is not an executive branch initiative but rather a congressional mandate. It has received a high level of attention in both the Senate and the House of Representatives.

The specific goal of GPRA is to focus agency and oversight attention on the outcomes of government activities—the results produced for the American public. The approach is to develop measures of outcomes that can be tied to annual budget allocations. To that end, the law requires each agency to produce three documents: a strategic plan, which sets general goals and objectives over a minimal 5-year period; a performance plan, which translates the goals of the strategic plan into annual targets; and a performance report, which demonstrates whether the targets were met. Agencies delivered the first required strategic plans to Congress in September 1997 and the first performance plans in the spring of 1998. Performance reports are due in March 2000. The law calls for strategic plans to be updated every 3 years and the other documents annually.

The general principles of GPRA have been implemented by many state governments and in other countries (for example, Canada, New Zealand, and the U.K.), but implementation by the U.S. federal government is the largest scale application of the concept to date and somewhat different. Over the last 5 years, various states have tried to develop performance measures of their investments. With respect to performance measures of science and technology activities, states tend to rely on an economic-development perspective with measures reflecting job creation and commercialization. Managers struggle to define appropriate measures, and level-of-activity measures dominate their assessments.[3] With respect to other countries, our limited review of their experiences showed that most are struggling with the same issues that the United States is concerned with, notably how to measure the results of basic research.

Not every aspect of the system worked perfectly the first time around in the United States. Some agencies started the learning process earlier and scaled up faster than others. OMB allowed considerable agency experimentation with different approaches to similar activities, waiting to see what ideas emerged. The expectations of and thus the guidance from the various congressional and executive audiences for strategic and performance plans have not always been the same and that has made it difficult for agencies to develop plans agreeable to all parties. Groups outside government that are likely to be interested in agency implementation of GPRA have not been consulted as extensively as envisioned. There is general agreement that all relevant parties should be engaged in a continuing learning process, and there are high expectations for improvement in future iterations.

The development of plans to implement GPRA has been particularly difficult for agencies responsible for research activities supported by the federal government. A report by GAO (GAO, 1997) indicates that measuring performance and results is particularly challenging for regulatory programs, scientific research programs, and programs that deliver services to taxpayers through third parties, such as state and local governments.

Findings from Workshops

From January through June 1998, COSEPUP held a series of workshops to gather information about the implementation of GPRA. The first workshop, cosponsored with the Academy Industry Program, focused on the approaches that industry uses to develop strategic plans and performance assessments. Industry participants emphasized the importance of having a strategic plan that clearly articulates the goals and objectives of the organization. One of the industry participants said that the objective of their industrial research is "knowledge generation with a purpose." The industry representative indicated that the company must first support world-class research programs that create new ideas; second, relate the new ideas to an important need within the organization or project; and third, build new competence in technologies and people. With respect to performance assessment, many industry participants noted that results of applied research and development programs are more easily quantified than results of basic research. However, even though they might not be able to quantify results of basic research, they nonetheless support it because they believe it important to their business; investments in basic research do pay off over time.[4]

With respect to assessing basic research, industry representatives indicated that they must rely on the judgment of individuals knowledgeable about the content of the research and the objectives of the organization to evaluate the results of such efforts. Some industry participants stressed the importance of giving careful consideration to any metrics one adopts—whether in industrial or government research. It is important to choose measures well and use them efficiently to minimize non-productive efforts. The metrics used also will change the behavior of the people being measured. For example, in basic research, if you measure relatively unimportant indicators, such as the number of publications per researcher instead of the quality of those publications, you will foster activities that may not be very productive or useful to the organization. A successful performance assessment program will both encourage positive behavior and discourage negative behavior. Metrics must be simple, not easily manipulated, and drive the right behavior. Most industry R&D metrics are more applicable to assessing applied research and technology development activities in the mission agencies.

The second COSEPUP workshop focused on the strategic and performance plans of 10 federal agencies: the Department of Defense, the Department of Energy, the Department of Transportation, the Department of Agriculture, the National Aeronautics and Space Administration, the National Institutes of Health, the National Science Foundation, the Environmental Protection Agency, the National Institute of Standards and Technology, and the National Oceanic and Atmospheric Administration. As might be expected, most of these organizations use different approaches to translate the goals in their strategic plans into performance goals for scientific and engineering research. Some agencies use qualitative, others quantitative, and still others, a combination of qualitative and quantitative measures. There was a strong consensus among the agencies that the practical outcomes of basic research cannot be captured by quantitative measures alone. Agency representatives generally agreed that progress in program management and facility operation can be assigned quantitative values.

Agencies with long-term targeted research goals have generally translated them into short-term milestones that can be achieved within a 2-year time horizon for performance planning and reporting. Agencies that seek advances in knowledge in broad fields rather than targeted ones, have not used the milestone approach to performance planning and reporting.

Some agencies have had difficulty in implementing GPRA. When preparing GPRA strategic and performance plans, some agencies are more likely than others to highlight research activities. The major variable is the magnitude of research relative to the agency's other activities. Submersion of research within large agencies makes it impossible for an integrated view of the federal science and technology investment to emerge through the GPRA process and is therefore a matter of concern for COSEPUP.

The performance plans of the agencies tend to emphasize short-term applied research with practical outcomes. Some participants expressed concern that this emphasis would skew funding away from long-term research that is difficult to measure against annual milestones.

Some participants indicated that a desirable result of GPRA would be to increase teamwork among the agencies, as well as to improve communication between research agencies and oversight entities, including Congress, OMB, and GAO. Another theme that recurred throughout the workshop was that the research community has a low level of awareness and is not strongly involved in the GPRA process.

The education and training of graduate and undergraduate students are among the most important duties and durable legacies of the research agencies. Yet human resources was not thoroughly identified or addressed in most agencies' performance plans.

Peer review was identified as the primary method for assessing the quality of research. However, the process by which peer review is applied varies widely among the agencies. Peer review of projects, grants, and contracts differs from peer review of programs and of intramural and extramural research. Those differences led COSEPUP to hold a third workshop focused on peer review and other methods for evaluating research.

In its third workshop, COSEPUP discussed the various methods available for evaluating research. As a result of that workshop and other discussions, COSEPUP found that the following methods are currently available for analyzing research:

1. Bibliometric analysis.
2. Economic rate of return.
3. Peer review.
4. Case study.
5. Retrospective analysis.
6. Benchmarking.

Each of these methods is briefly described below.[5] The pros and cons associated with each technique are summarized in Table 1, later in this chapter.

Bibliometric Analysis[6]

A technique known as bibliometric analysis, which includes publications, citations, and patent counts, is based on the premise that a researcher's work has value when it is judged by peers to have merit. A manuscript is published in a refereed journal only when expert reviewers and the editor approve its quality; a published work is cited by other researchers as recognition of its authority; and a published work is cited as evidence by a company applying for a patent. By extension, the more times a work is cited, the greater its merit. The primary benefit of bibliometric analysis is its quantitative nature. Furthermore, it correlates well (approximately 60% in one study) with peer review when both methods are used.

The primary argument against bibliometric anaylsis is that bibliometric measurements treat all citations as equally important. However, many citations refer to routine methods or statistical designs, modifications of techniques, or standard data or even refute the validity of a paper. Other problems are caused by citing the first-named author of a publication when the customs that determine the order in which authors are listed vary by fields. In

TABLE 1: CURRENT METHODS USED FOR EVALUATING RESEARCH

Methods	**Pro**	**Con**
Bibliometric analysis	Quantitative; useful on aggregate basis to evaluate quality for some programs and fields	At best, measures only quantity; not useful across all programs & fields; comparisons across fields or countries difficult; can be artificially influenced
Economic rate of return	Quantitative; shows economic benefits of research	Measures only financial benefits, not social benefits (such as health-quality improvements); time separating research from economic benefit is often long; not useful across all programs and fields
Peer review	Well-understood method and practices; provides evaluation of quality of research and sometimes other factors; already an existing part of most federal-agency programs in evaluating the quality of research projects	Focuses primarily on research quality; other elements are secondary; evaluation usually of research projects, not programs; great variance across agencies; concerns regarding use of "old boy network"; results depend on involvement of high-quality people in process
Case studies	Provides understanding of effects of institutional, organizational, and technical factors influencing research process, so process can be improved; illustrates all types of benefits of research process	Happenstance cases not comparable across programs; focus on cases that might involve many programs or fields making it difficult to assess federal-program benefit
Retrospective analysis	Useful for identifying linkages between federal programs and innovations over long intervals of research investment	Not useful as a short-term evaluation tool because of long interval between research and practical outcomes
Benchmarking	Provides a tool for comparison across programs and countries	Focused on fields, not federal research programs

addition, different mores among research communities—whether particular disciplines or countries—can skew results when they are used comparatively (for example, far fewer outlets are available for Russian publications than for U.S. publications). Furthermore, in emphasizing counts, researchers are apt to take actions that artificially increase the number of citations they receive or reduce their research in fields that offer less opportunity of immediate or frequent publication or in critical related fields (such as education) that do not offer publication opportunities.

Economic Rate of Return

In recent years, economists have developed a number of techniques to estimate the economic benefits (such as rate of return) of research. The primary benefit of this method is that it provides a metric of research outcomes. However, there are a number of difficulties. In particular, the American Enterprise Institute (AEI, 1994) found that existing economic methods and data are sufficient to measure only a subset of important dimensions of the outcomes and impacts of fundamental science. Economic methods are best suited to assessing mission-agency programs and less-well suited to assessing the work of fundamental research agencies, particularly on an annual basis. Furthermore, economists are not able to estimate the benefit-to-cost ratio "at the margin" for fundamental science (that is, the marginal rate of return—or how much economic benefit is received for an additional dollar investment in research), and it is this information that is needed to make policy decisions. Finally, the time that separates the research from its ultimate beneficial outcome is often very long—50-some years is not unusual.

Peer Review[7]

Peer review is the method by which science exercises continuous self-evaluation and correction. It is the centerpiece of many federal agencies' approach to evaluating proposed, current, and past research in science and engineering.

Peer review, like all human judgments, can be affected by self-interest, especially the favoritism of friendship and the prejudice of antagonism. However, those distortions can be minimized by the rigor of peer selection, the integrity and independence of individual reviewers, and the use of bibliometric analysis and other quantitative techniques to complement the subjective nature of peer review.

Peer review is not equally appropriate across the wide span of research performed by federal agencies. We might visualize at one end of the spectrum the fundamental, long-term projects whose ultimate outcomes are unpredictable and at the other end programs of incremental or developmental work whose results are easier to predict within fairly narrow time limits. Projects of the latter type can often be evaluated in a rigorously quantifiable fashion by appropriate metrics. It is for the former kind of research, whose results are not easily quantified, especially while the work is in progress, that peer review of quality and leadership is required and generally effective. Agency managers have the responsibility of designing review techniques that suit the nature of each individual research program being evaluated.

Case Studies

Historical accounts of the social and intellectual developments that led to key events in science or applications of science illuminate the discovery process in greater depth than other methods. The chief advantage of case studies is that they can be used to understand the effects of institutional, organizational, and technical factors on the research process and can identify important outcomes of the research process that are not purely intellectual, such as the collaboration of other researchers, the training of young researchers, and the development of productive research centers.

Difficulties of case studies are that they can be expensive, and that the validity of the results and conclusions depends on the objectivity, investigative skills, and scientific knowledge of the persons doing them.

Retrospective Analysis

Retrospective analyses are related to case studies in that they also try to reconstruct history; however, they focus on multiple scientific or technological innovations rather than just one. The goal is to identify linkages between innovations and particular types of antecedent events (usually either funding or research). Such analysis is usually done by a panel of experts or investigators. This method is most appropriate for assessing a particular type of accountability question (for example, impact of National Science Foundation funding on mathematics research). The primary disadvantage of this type of analysis is that it takes a long time to conduct and thus is not useful as a tool to provide short-term evaluations for improving research policy and management.

Benchmarking[8]

As noted earlier, maintaining leadership across the frontiers of science is a critical element of the nation's investment strategy for research (COSEPUP, 1993). The question addressed here is, whether an agency's or the nation's research and educational programs are at the cutting edge? This assessment is made by a panel of international and national academic and industrial experts in a given field and in related fields on the basis of available quantitative and qualitative data. COSEPUP has conducted a number of experimental efforts on benchmarking the United States' position in selected fields. Programs can be benchmarked in a similar fashion.

NOTES

3. For more information regarding individual states see http://www.gsu.edu/~padjem/projects.html.[G-14]

4. For additional information on corporate experience in assessing research and its applicablity to federal research, see Commission on Physical Sciences, Mathematics, and Applications, (1995) Research Restructuring and Assessment, National Academy Press, Washington, D.C.

5. These descriptions were adapted from the National Science and Technology Council's (NSTC) Assessing Fundamental Science, 1996.

6. Small, Henry G. "A Co-Citation Model of a Scientific Specialty: A Longitudinal Study of Collagen Research" Social Studies of Science Vol. 7 (1977), 139-66. Anderson, Richard C., F. Narin, Paul McAllister "Publication Ratings versus Peer Ratings of Universities" Journal of the American Society for Information Science March (1978) 91-103.

7. For additional information on peer review, see Atkinson, Richard C. and William A. Blanpied, Peer Review and the Public Interest, Issues in Science and Technology, vol 1. no. 4, 1985; Bozeman, B. and J. Melkers, "Peer Review and Evaluation of R&D Impacts," Evaluating R&D Impacts, Kluwer Academic Publishers, Norwell, Mass., (1993) 79-98; Cole, J. and S. Cole, Peer Review in the National Science Foundation, Washington, D.C.: National Academy Press, 1981; GAO, Peer Review; Reforms Needed to Ensure Fairness in Federal Agency Grant Selection, June 1984.

8. See COSEPUP, 1997 and COSEPUP, 1998.

CHAPTER 2

RESEARCH AND THE FEDERAL GOVERNMENT

Results of Federal Investment in Research

The nation benefits from its investment in federal research in four major ways: knowledge advancement, knowledge application, human capital development, and mission advancement. It is important that all four of these be considered when evaluating the federal investment in research.

Knowledge advancement lays the basis of our understanding of nature, which can later be built on for practical outcomes. Furthermore, it leads to better awareness and understanding of the world and universe around us and our place therein, as was the case when the Hubble telescope began transmitting pictures from the farthest reaches of space.

Knowledge application is capitalizing on research to produce economic or societal benefits. In some cases, new research discoveries have led to new categories of industry, such as the fast-growing industries that have emerged from research in information technology and biotechnology. In other cases, society reaps the benefits of research in the form of public-health improvements, a sound defense, or a cleaner environment.

Human capital development is a key outcome of the research process that is often overlooked. The ability of the nation to respond to societal needs is related directly to the human skills required to address particular problems. The federal government supports, directly through grants, loans, or fellowships or indirectly through campus research, the people who are educated in the nation's undergraduate and graduate education system and who enter professions in all sectors of society. Government and industry both support continuing education for scientists and engineers who want to sharpen their skills and acquire new ones. These people constitute the best mechanism for transferring knowledge from teachers and researchers in higher education to business, government, education, and other institutions. A key aspect of a student's educational experience is working with researchers who are supported by the federal government; alternatively, graduate and postdoctoral researchers receive fellowship funds directly via the research that they conduct under the guidance of a mentor. The outcome of this process is a new generation of knowledgeable people capable of addressing societal problems. Our federal laboratories also train personnel who can contribute to agency missions and to private-sector activity.

Finally, the nation benefits as agencies strive to meet their objectives. *Mission advancement* is an outcome that is specific to particular mission agencies. Each agency has a particular mission that is linked to societal objectives, such as improving the environment, developing new forms of energy, probing the universe, developing new technologies, improving the health of our people, and providing for the national defense. And each agency funds research—both basic and applied—that is intended to accomplish its particular mission and thus achieve societal goals. The results can be as varied as discovering a new planet, reducing the cost of energy, and developing techniques of warfare that require fewer personnel.

Goals of Federal Investment in Research

Given the variety of research supported by the federal government and the outcomes of its investment, what are the appropriate goals for agencies that support research? In its 1993 report *Science, Technology, and the Federal Government: National Goals for a New Era*, COSEPUP discussed this issue and made the following recommendation:

The United States should be among the world leaders in all major fields of science.

COSEPUP based that recommendation on several observations. First, it is impossible to predict the ultimate practical outcomes of scientific research. For example, basic research on electromagnetism in the 19th century led to the development of modern communication in the 20th century; research in quantum physics 5 decades ago, followed by research in solid-state physics, led to the transistor and semiconductor electronics; and studies of unusual enzymes in bacteria led to recombinant-DNA technology and then to the modern biotechnology industry. None of those outcomes was directly expected by those who performed the basic research. Today, COSEPUP would extend that recommendation to include basic research in engineering.

Second, and in the same vein, it is important to perform sound research for which applications are not yet known. The motivation of researchers who conduct basic research, primarily in universities, might or might not be the desire to develop new applications; many researchers are motivated primarily by the desire to discover and to understand the basic workings of nature. But funders who understand the workings of the research process know that investments in excellent research in important fields of science and engineering have, in the aggregate, enormous payoffs in terms of practical outcomes.

Finally, the United States has risen to a position of global prominence because of numerous factors, including natural resources, political stability, economic freedom, and strength in science and engineering. Strength in science and engineering can and must continue to contribute to U.S. leadership. Being among the leaders in each field of science and engineering means that U.S. scientists and engineers can understand, participate in, and capitalize on the expansion of the frontiers of human knowledge.

COSEPUP made a second, complementary recommendation for U.S. science policy:

The United States should maintain clear leadership in selected fields of science.

Again, COSEPUP would amend that to include engineering research. The selection of fields for clear world leadership should be informed by scientific and engineering input but in the end should generally rest on societal judgment, not a scientific judgment. It is a judgment that money spent to obtain clear leadership will give a large societal return. That return could be in providing industry leadership (as in molecular biology) or in a rapid advance in our ability to deal with diseases, or in a contribution to a better environment—whatever it is that our society values and in which clear world leadership would make a difference.

The fields in which clear leadership is a goal should be defined by government policy-makers in close collaboration with interested groups, including especially the generators and users of science and technology. Policy-makers should be fully informed of the comparative assessments of the U.S. position in scientific fields (by international benchmarking). Choosing fields in which the United States should maintain clear leadership is a different kind of process from deciding on the most promising directions for research in a given field of science or engineering.

MEASURING AND EVALUATING FEDERALLY FUNDED RESEARCH

Measuring Research

The unique characteristics of research activities, particularly those whose ultimate practical outcomes cannot be known, present challenges to research agencies seeking to implement GPRA, but COSEPUP believes that research programs, no matter what their character and goals, can be evaluated meaningfully on a regular basis in accordance with the spirit and intent of GPRA. To accomplish that evaluation, methods must be chosen to match the character of the research. Results of applied research can often be evaluated in quantitative terms according to specific timelines; basic research in science and engineering cannot always be evaluated in quantitative terms but can be assessed against carefully designed measures that serve as guides to research direction, funding allocations, and policy decisions.

In applied research programs of mission agencies, specific practical outcomes can be documented and progress evaluated annually. For example, if the Department of Energy (DOE) adopted the goal of producing cheaper solar energy, it could measure the results of research designed to decrease the cost of solar cells. In this situation, an applied research program can be evaluated against specific measurable milestones annually. Other programs that could be evaluated in similar fashion are efforts to build an optical computer, breed drought-resistant or saline-tolerant crops, assemble a prototype for a walking robot, devise a prototype DNA-sequencing machine, use vitrification for storage of nuclear and hazardous waste, and adapt fiber-optic laser surgery for treatment of prostatic cancer.

Speech Recognition

Many long-term research programs proceed in the anticipation of a known, desired outcome. In the case of speech recognition, for example, the known, desired outcome is the development of computers that can "understand" and act on the spoken word with a high degree of accuracy. It is impossible to predict when the goal will be reached, partly because of the many technical hurdles that must be overcome: people have different accents, words can be slurred or mispronounced; languages contain hidden grammatical traps, and the voices of multiple speakers need to be differentiated.

In measuring the results of speech-recognition research, it is important to understand the step-by-step process by which hurdles must be overcome. The long-term achievement of desired outcomes can be divided into separate research efforts, each of which has its own performance level that can be targeted and measured annually to demonstrate progress. For example, in regard to speech recognition, all the following can be quantified: the size and extent of a program's vocabulary; the rate at which a speaker must talk, the length of pauses needed between words; accuracy rates for different accents and pronunciations; and the ability to punctuate, choose between homonyms, and spell unknown words.

Basic research programs can be evaluated meaningfully on a regular basis, but as explained in Chapter 2, ultimate outcomes of research into fundamental processes are seldom predictable or quantifiable in advance. It is normal and necessary for basic research investigators to modify their goals, change course, and test competing hypotheses as they move closer to the fundamental understandings that justify public investment in their work. Therefore, it is necessary to evaluate the performance of basic-research programs by using measures not of practical outcomes but of performance, such as the generation of new knowledge, the quality of research, the attainment of leadership in the field, and the development of human resources.

Historical evidence shows us unmistakably that by any measure, the benefit of leadership in science and engineering to the United States is extremely high. Many agree on this point.[10]

History also shows us how often basic research leads to outcomes that were unexpected or whose emergence took place over many years or even decades after the basic research was performed. For example, pre-World War II basic studies of research on atomic structure contributed, after decades of work, to today's Global Positioning System, an outcome of great practical and economic value. Attempts to evaluate a year's worth of that early research would have contained no hint of this particular outcome, but annual evaluations would have demonstrated the continuing high quality of the research being performed and continuing U.S. leadership in the field—a result that is traditionally followed by great practical, intellectual, and economic benefits.

Investing in Basic Research: Atomic Physics

Federal investments in basic research can sustain long-term work that can lead to technologies unimagined when the research was initiated. It was impossible to guess the far-reaching ramifications of I.I. Rabi's research on molecular-beam magnetic resonance in the late 1930s or Norman Ramsey's invention of a separated oscillatory-field resonance method in 1949. Yet the research of Rabi and Ramsey constitute the scientific basis for modern-day atomic clocks (accurate to within 1 second in 100,000 years) and global positioning systems (GPS).

With the declassification of the GPS in 1993, this grandchild of atomic physics has become an innovation of great economic and practical importance. Installed in automobiles, GPS can tell drivers not only where they are, but how to get to their destination. Thanks to the GPS, soldiers stranded behind enemy lines can be rescued with surgical precision; backpackers, firefighters, and people in sailboats, crop-dusters, and automobiles can all be confident of their exact location. The worldwide market for positioning systems is expected to surpass $30 billion in the next decade.

Annual evaluations of quality and leadership give a strong indication of the likelihood of important long-term practical outcomes of basic research, but a historical review can provide reality.

Not every specific basic research program can be expected to have a practical outcome, so the backward look must extend over a diverse array of programs. Also, because the interval between basic research progress and practical outcomes can be decades, the view back must also be long. It should not consist of asking for the practical outcomes of research conducted in the previous year.

Federal agencies support a great number of long-term investigations that have extremely valuable outcomes that are unknown at the start of the investigations. These projects include explorations of the evolution of the universe, of the chemistry of photosynthesis, of the dynamics of plate tectonics, of the composition of Earth's core, and of how language is acquired. The appropriate measure of each such programs is the quality, relevance, and leadership of the research.

Using Expert Review to Evaluate Research Programs

Because of the nature of the research process, assessing its results requires an evaluation technique of breadth and flexibility. During the course of this study, COSEPUP assessed a number of methods used to evaluate research, including economic-impact studies, citation analyses, and patent analyses. Each of those methodologies might have merit, but COSEPUP concluded that they do not provide the rigor of expert review (although when appropriate they should be used by experts to complement their review). For example, economic-impact studies conducted annually are useful for applied research but inappropriate for basic research, although they can be useful in the retrospective review of the practical outcomes of basic research; citation analyses require expert evaluation of the content, quality, and relevance of citations; patent analyses also can provide useful information, especially in applied research programs, but require expert evaluation of patent quality and relevance. COSEPUP recognizes the legitimate concerns that have been raised about expert review (such as conflict of interest, independence, and elitism) but believes that, when implemented with careful planning and design, various kinds of expert review are the most rigorous and effective tools for evaluating basic and applied research.

The best-known form of expert review is *peer review*, developed from the premise that a scientist's or engineer's peers have the essential knowledge and perspective to judge the quality of research and are the best qualified people to do so. Peer review is commonly used to make many kinds of judgments: about the careers of individual researchers, about the value of their publications, about the standing of research institutions, and about the allocation of funds to individuals and to fields of research (COSEPUP, 1982).

A second form of expert review is *relevance review*, in which a panel is composed of potential users of the results of research, experts in fields related to the field of research, and scientists or engineers from the field itself. The goal of relevance review is to judge whether an agency's research programs are relevant to its mission. Expert researchers are essential to this process because of their perspective on the field and their knowledge of other research projects in the field or in similar fields. Relevance review should not be confined to applied research, in which desired outcomes are defined. Relevance review should also consider basic research projects funded by federal agencies. Although the ultimate practical outcomes of basic research cannot be predicted, it is important to ascertain whether a given line of research is likely to contribute to an agency's mission. For example, if a goal of DOE is to produce cheaper solar energy, it is consistent with the agency's mission to understand the physical properties that determine the ability of materials to convert solar radiation into electrical energy. A careful relevance review could indicate the most promising directions for future research, both basic and applied.

A third form of expert review is *benchmarking*, which evaluates the relative international standing of U.S. research efforts. International benchmarking by panels of international experts evaluates the relative leadership among nations in fields of science and engineering. Benchmarking exercises have already been conducted by COSEPUP (in mathematics, material science and engineering, and immunology) and by the National Science Foundation (in mathematics). Those exercises have demonstrated that benchmarking can be an effective means of determining leadership in a field. Although the principal reliance is on the judgment of experts, quantitative measures can also be used for confirmation.

Leadership positions in fields of science and engineering are a result of substantial infrastructures of people and facilities built over several years; they generally do not shift annually. Thus, international benchmarking reviews, every few years, can provide adequate information. Agencies can still report annually on the U.S. leadership position by observing major discoveries or other changes that have occurred in the preceding year. Important changes can occur whenever programs are being dismantled or reduced. The impact of these reductions on U.S. leadership positions should be noted in annual reports.

Assembling a panel of people who have sufficient breadth and depth to make sound assessments is the responsibility of agency management. The competence and dedication of review managers can substantially enhance the value of reviews. Expert review is not effective without proper planning and guidance, and it should always be viewed as a management tool rather than as a substitute for vision, planning, and decision-making.

Enhancing the Expert Review Process

Because of the great variation in structure and mission of federal agencies that support research, the ways in which various agencies review their research will inevitably differ. Each agency must develop the approach that serves best as a management and reporting vehicle. However, additional actions can enhance the implementation of GPRA to the mutual benefit of agencies and communities that provide or depend on agency funding.

It is common and useful for multiple agencies to approach similar fields of research from different perspectives. Indeed, such pluralism is a major strength of the U.S. research enterprise. However, better communication among agencies would enhance opportunities for collaboration, help prevent important questions from being overlooked, and reduce instances of inefficient duplication of effort. According to the comments in our workshops, present coordination mechanisms need strengthening.

The review process could be made more effective through the greater involvement of the research community at large. COSEPUP members, on the basis of their own experience and of the workshops and research conducted for this report, have been struck by the small number of researchers who are aware of the intent of GPRA and its relevance and importance both to their work and to the procedures of federal agencies that support research. The researchers who work in agency, university, and industrial laboratories are the people who perform and best understand the research funded by the federal government. The research community should be involved in developing the processes that agencies will use to measure and evaluate the results of research. The agencies should encourage comment from the research community. Members of the research community also must be part of the expert-review process of measuring and evaluating results of research programs. The research community is essential to measuring and evaluating quality, leadership, and, in some cases, relevance of research programs.

Summary

COSEPUP believes that results of federal research programs can be evaluated meaningfully on a regular basis in accordance with the spirit and intent of GPRA. However, the methods of evaluation must be chosen to match the character of research and its objectives. Furthermore, the committee believes that expert review is the most effective mechanism for evaluating the quality, leadership, and relevance of research (especially basic research) performed and funded by federal agencies. Ultimately, decisions regarding the selection and funding of research programs must be made by agency managers informed by expert review.

NOTE

10. See Landau, Ralph, Technology, Economics, and Public Policy. In Landau, Ralph and Dale W. Jorgensen, eds. Technology and Economic Policy. Cambridge, Ballinger Publ. Co., 1986; Carnegie Commission on Science, Technology, and Government. Enabling the Future: Linking Science and Technology to Societal Goals (Carnegie Commission: New York, NY 1992); Nadiri, M. Ishaq. "Innovations and Technological Spillovers," Working Paper No. 4423 (National Bureau of Economic Research: Cambridge, MA, August 1993).

CHAPTER 4

RECOMMENDATIONS

Federal agencies that support research in science and engineering have been challenged to find the most useful and effective ways to evaluate the performance and results of research programs that they support. Through a series of workshops and panel discussions involving industry, agency, and oversight personnel, COSEPUP has gathered information and formulated principles that can be helpful to agencies in evaluating their research programs and helpful to oversight bodies in considering the evaluations. COSEPUP offers six recommendations. COSEPUP intends to address mechanisms and guidelines for implementing the recommendations in meetings and workshops with representatives from agencies and congressional and other oversight bodies. Given the diverse portfolio of research conducted by federal agencies and the urgency of addressing the questions of how research can be evaluated in the context of GPRA, the level of detail and specificity needed in designing procedures and guidelines for implementation was beyond the scope of this report.

Recommendation 1: Because both applied research and basic research can be evaluated meaningfully on a regular basis and are vital to research and mission agencies, research programs should be described in strategic and performance plans and evaluated in performance reports.

The performance of research is critical to the missions of many federal agencies. Therefore, a full description of an agency's goals and results, which is a principal objective of GPRA, must contain an evaluation of research activities and their relevance to the agency's mission.

Recommendation 2: For applied research programs, agencies should measure progress toward practical outcomes. For basic research programs, agencies should measure quality, relevance, and leadership. In addition, agencies should conduct periodic reviews of the overall practical outcomes of an agency's overall past support of applied and basic research. The use of measurements needs to recognize what can and cannot be measured. Misuse of measurement can lead to strongly negative results; for example, measuring basic research on the basis of short-term relevance would be extremely destructive to quality work.

Because the evaluation of applied research is directly connected to practical outcomes, whereas the evaluation of basic research is in terms of quality, relevance, and leadership, which ultimately lead to practical outcomes, there might be a tendency to bias an agency's overall research program toward applied research at the expense of basic research. This should be avoided, and a proper balance should be maintained.

Recommendation 3: Federal agencies should use expert review to assess the quality of research they support, the relevance of that research to their mission, and the leadership of the research. Expert review must strive for balance between having the most knowledgeable and the most independent individuals serve as members. Each agency should develop clear, explicit guidance with regard to structuring and employing expert review processes.

The most effective way to evaluate research programs is by expert review. The most commonly used form of expert review of quality is peer review. This operates on the premise that the people best qualified to judge the quality of research are experts in the field of research. This premise prevails across the research spectrum, from basic research to applied research. A second form of expert review is relevance review, in which potential users and experts in other fields or disciplines related to an agency's mission or to the potential application of the research evaluate the relevance of research to the agency's mission. A third form of expert review is benchmarking, in which an international panel of experts compares the level of leadership of a research program relative to research being performed worldwide.

Recommendation 4: Both research and mission agencies should describe in their strategic and performance plans the goal of developing and maintaining adequate human resources in fields critical to their missions both at the national level and in their agencies. Human resources should become a part of the evaluation of a research program along with the program's quality in terms of research advancement, relevance in terms of application development, and leadership in terms of the ability to take advantage of opportunities when they arise.

In early drafts of strategic and performance plans, agencies have generally omitted discussions of education and training, which are fundamental to the ability of agencies to fulfill their missions. The goal of developing and maintaining adequate human resources in fields critical to their missions should be supported by plans that produce that outcome. The nation cannot benefit from advances in science and technology without a continuing supply of well-educated and well-trained scientists and engineers. In addition, in the absence of such a flow, the capability of an agency to fulfill its mission will be compromised and the knowledge learned and technology developed will be lost.

Recommendation 5: Although GPRA is conducted agency-by-agency, a formal process should be established to identify and coordinate areas of research that are supported by multiple agencies. A lead agency should be identified for each field of research and that agency should be responsible for assuring that coordination occurs among the agencies.

It is common and valuable for multiple agencies to approach similar fields of research from different perspectives. Indeed, this pluralism is a major strength of the U.S. research enterprise. However, better communication among agencies would enhance opportunities for collaboration, help to keep important questions from being overlooked, and reduce instances of inefficient duplication of effort. A single agency should be identified to serve as the focal point for each particular field of research so that all significant supported fields are covered. Information regarding support for that field should be provided to all the agencies involved in it so that they can adjust their efforts to ensure that the field is appropriately covered. Agencies should use benchmarking, which affords the opportunity to look across fields, in their efforts to understand the status of a particular field of research.

Recommendation 6: The science and engineering community can and should play an important role in GPRA implementation. As a first step, they should become familiar with agency strategic and performance plans, which are available on the agencies' web sites.

The researchers who work in agency, university, and industrial laboratories are the people who perform and best understand the research programs funded by the federal government.

Many researchers contribute substantial time and effort to reviewing papers submitted for publication, grant applications, and program proposals, but few of them are aware of GPRA. Their greater involvement in implementing GPRA would be beneficial to the country. Increased contact with and advice from the broader scientific and engineering community regarding both the quality and the leadership position of agency research programs and the relevance of the research to agency missions can benefit the GPRA process.

COMMITTEE ON SCIENCE, ENGINEERING, AND PUBLIC POLICY

MEMBERS' BIOGRAPHICAL INFORMATION

Committee Chair

Phillip A. Griffiths has been Director of the Institute for Advanced Study since 1991. He was the Provost and James B. Duke Professor of Mathematics of Duke University from 1983-1991. In 1983 he was the Dwight Parker Robinson Professor of Mathematics at Harvard University. Phillip, a member of the National Science Board, became a member of the National Academy of Sciences in 1979. He chaired the Board on Mathematical Sciences from 1986-91, and Commission on Physical Sciences, Mathematics, and Applications in 1992. He was the recipient of the LeRoy Steele Prize given by the American Mathematical Society, and Dannie Heineman Prize of the Academy of Sciences at Gottingen.

Bruce M. Alberts, President of the National Academy of Sciences, is a respected biochemist recognized for his work in both biochemistry and molecular biology. He is noted particularly for his extensive study of the protein complexes that allow chromosomes to be replicated, as required for a living cell to divide. Bruce is a past Chair of the Commission on Life Sciences. He has served on the faculties of Princeton University, and as Vice Chair and Chair of the UCSF Department of Biochemistry and Biophysics. Being committed to the improvement of science education, he has dedicated much of his time to education projects in San Francisco elementary schools.

Peter Diamond is an Institute Professor at the Massachusetts Institute of Technology, where he has taught since 1966. He received his B.A. in Mathematics from Yale University in 1960 and his Ph.D. in Economics from MIT in 1963. He is Chair of the Board of the National Academy of Social Insurance, where he has been President. He has been President of the Econometric Society and Vice-President of the American Economic Association. He is a Fellow of the American Academy of Arts and Sciences, a Member of the National Academy of Sciences, and a Founding Member of the National Academy of Social Insurance. He was the recipient of the 1980 Mahalanobis Memorial Award and the 1994 Nemmers Prize. He has written on public finance, social insurance, uncertainty and search theories, and the macroeconomics.

Gerald P. Dinneen was Foreign Secretary of the National Academy of Engineering from 1988 until 1995. He was previously Vice President of Science and Technology at Honeywell Corporation and from 1977-81 he was the Assistant Secretary of Defense and Principal Deputy Under Secretary of Defense for Research and Engineering. He has had a long affiliation with the Massachusetts Institute of Technology since 1953 when he joined the MIT Lincoln Laboratory in Lexington, MA. He advanced through many positions to become the Director, 1970-77, and concurrently, a Professor of Electrical Engineering, 1971-81. He was elected to the National Academy of Engineering in 1975 and serves on many advisory committees and boards for the National Research Council and in government. He has been elected to the Engineering Academy of Japan, the Swiss Academy of Technological Sciences, and the Royal Academy of Engineering of the U.K.

Mildred S. Dresselhaus is currently the Institute Professor of Electrical Engineering and Physics at the Massachusetts Institute of Technology, where she held the Abby Rockefeller Mauze Chair at MIT in Electrical Engineering and in Physics, and directed the Center for Materials Science and Engineering. She has been active in the study of a wide range of problems in the physics of solids, and the modification of the properties of electronic materials by intercalation and implantation, the structure and properties of carbon fibers, of fullerenes and carbon nanotubes, and of high T-c superconductors. She was awarded the National Medal of Science in November 1990, was elected to the National Academy of Engineering in 1974, and to the National Academy of Sciences in 1985. She has been a member of both Councils of NAE and NAS, the Governing Board, and has served on numerous committees including Chair of the Committee on Women in Science and Engineering, and has served as NAS Treasurer since 1992.

James J. Duderstadt is President Emeritus and University Professor of Science and Engineering at the University of Michigan. He received his B.A. from Yale University in 1964 and his doctorate in engineering science and physics from the California Institute of Technology in 1967. He joined the faculty of the University of Michigan in 1968 and has served as Professor of Nuclear Engineering, Dean of the College of Engineering, and then as Provost and Vice President for Academic Affairs. He was elected President of the University of Michigan in 1988 and served in that role until July 1996. He received the National Medal of Technology for exemplary service to the nation, the E.O. Lawrence Award for excellence in nuclear research, and the Arthur Holly Compton Prize for outstanding teaching. He has served as chair of the National Science Board, chair of the Board of Directors of the Big Ten Athletic Conference and chair of the Executive Board of the University of Michigan's Hospitals. He also serves as a director of the Unisys Corporation and CMS Energy Corporation. He has been a member of the National Academy of Engineering since 1987.

Marye Anne Fox, a chemist and member of the National Academy of Sciences, is North Carolina State University's 12th chancellor. Appointed on April 9, 1998, Marye Anne assumed the duties of the top post at the state's flagship science and technology university on August 1, 1998. Before this appointment, Marye

Anne was the M. June and J. Virgil Waggoner Regents Chair in Chemistry and Vice President for Research at the University of Texas at Austin. Her research interests include physical organic chemistry; organic photochemistry; organic electrochemistry; chemical reactivity in non-homogeneous systems; heterogeneous photocatalysis; and electronic transfer in anisotropic macromolecular arrays. Marye Anne currently serves on the Council of the NAS, its Executive Committee, and the Committee on Science and Education Policy. After U.S. Senate confirmation in 1990 of her nomination to the National Science Board, she served as its Vice Chairman (1994-96) and chaired its Committee on Programs and Plans (1991-94). She serves on the Texas Governor's Science and Technology Council, has chaired the Chemistry Section of AAAS, and advises its Center for Science, Technology and the Congress. She has served on advisory panels for the Army, the Department of Energy, the National Science Foundation, and the National Institutes of Health. She has served on 14 editorial boards, including a stint as associate editor of the *Journal of the American Chemical Society*. She serves on boards of the Texas Environmental Defense Fund, Texas Agribusiness Council, Texas Food and Fiber Commission, W.R. Grace, and Oak Ridge Associated Universities.

Ralph E. Gomory has been President of the Alfred P. Sloan Foundation since 1989. Following his university position as Higgins Lecturer and Assistant Professor at Princeton, he joined IBM in 1959, becoming Vice President in 1973, and Senior Vice President for Science and Technology from 1985-1989. A member of both the NAS and NAE, he has received the Lanchester Prize in 1963, the John von Neumann Theory Prize in 1984, the IEEE Engineering Leadership Recognition Award in 1988, and National Medal of Science in 1988. In 1990, he was named to the President's Council of Advisors on Science and Technology.

Ruby P. Hearn is senior vice president of The Robert Wood Johnson Foundation, the largest health care philanthropy in the

United States. The Foundation has awarded over two billion dollars in grant funds since its inception as a national philanthropy in 1972. As a member of the executive management team, Ruby participates in strategic program planning with the president and executive vice president and serves as a special advisor to the president and as the Foundation's liaison within the non-profit community. Dr. Hearn has had the major responsibility for oversight and program development of initiatives in maternal, infant and child health, AIDS, substance abuse and minority medical education. She received her MS and PhD degrees in biophysics from Yale University and is a graduate of Skidmore College. She is a Fellow, Yale Corporation. She served on the Executive Committee of the Board of Directors for the 1995 Special Olympics World Summer games in Connecticut, among others. She is a member of the Institute of Medicine and its governing Council, the National Academy of Sciences Committee on Science, Engineering, and Public Policy (COSEPUP), the Board of Directors of the Council on Foundations and the Science Board for the Food and Drug Administration (FDA), and is also serving on the Advisory Committee to the Director, National Institutes of Health.

Philip W. Majerus has been Co-Director of the Division of Hematology-Oncology at the Washington University School of Medicine since 1973. He holds concurrent positions as Professor of Biochemistry and Professor of Medicine at the Washington University School of Medicine, as Chairman of the James S. McDonnell Foundation's Program for Molecular Medicine in Cancer Research, as Chairman of NAS Section 41, Medical Genetics, Hematology and Oncology, and as Chairman of the Board of Scientific Advisors NHLBI. He was Chairman of the Searle Scholars Program (1989-1993), President of the American Society of Clinical Investigation (1981-1982) and of the American Society of Hematology (1991). Philip is an NAS and IOM member and is a Fellow with the American College of Physicians, the American Academy of Arts and

Sciences, and the American Association for the Advancement of Science. He is on the editorial board of the *Proceedings of the National Academy of Sciences*.

June E. Osborn is the sixth president of the Josiah Macy, Jr. Foundation in New York. She received a B.A. from Oberlin College in 1957 and an M.D. from Case Western Reserve University in 1961. She spent three years in training as a pediatric resident at Boston Children's and Massachusetts General Hospitals and then two years as a postdoctoral fellow in virology and infectious diseases at Johns Hopkins Medical School and at the University of Pittsburgh. From 1966 to 1984 she was on the faculty of the University of Wisconsin Medical School where she was Professor in the Departments of Medical Microbiology and of Pediatrics. In 1975 she also became Associate Dean for Biological Sciences in the University of Wisconsin Graduate School.

Kenneth I. Shine is President of the Institute of Medicine, and Professor of Medicine Emeritus at the University of California, Los Angeles School of Medicine. He is UCLA School of Medicine's immediate past Dean and Provost for Medical Services. He was Director of the Coronary Care Unit, Chief of the Cardiology Division, and Chair of the Department of Medicine at the UCLA School of Medicine. He has served as Chairman of the Council of Deans of the AAMC, and was President of the American Heart Association. His research interests include metabolic events in the heart muscle, the relation of behavior to heart disease, and emergency medicine.

Morris Tanenbaum was the Vice Chairman of the Board and Chief Financial Officer of AT&T from 1988-1991. He began his career at Bell Telephone Labs on the technical staff, held various positions at Western Electric Company including Vice President of the Engineering Division and Vice President of Manufacturing, before returning to Bell Labs in 1975 as Executive Vice President.

In 1978 he became President of New Jersey Bell Telephone Company, returned to AT&T as Executive Vice President, Corporate Affairs and Planning in 1980, becoming the first Chairman and CEO of AT&T Communications in 1984. Morry was Vice President of NAE until June 1998.

William Julius Wilson is the Malcolm Wiener Professor of Social Policy at the John F. Kennedy School of Government, Harvard University. He was formerly Lucy Flower University Professor of Sociology and Public Policy at the University of Chicago. He is a member of the National Academy of Sciences, the American Academy of Arts and Sciences, the National Academy of Education, and former member of the President's Committee on the National Medal of Science, and past President of both the American Sociological Association and the Consortium of Social Science Associations (COSSA).

William A. Wulf is President of NAE. The former NAE Councillor, he was AT&T Professor of Engineering and Applied Science at the University of Virginia. He has served as Assistant Director of the National Science Foundation, Chairman and CEO of Tartan Laboratories, Inc., and as Professor of Computer Science at Carnegie Mellon University. He has been a member of NAE since 1993, and serves as Chair of the Computer Science and Telecommunications Board.

Staff

Richard Bissell is Executive Director of the Policy Division and Director of COSEPUP. He took up his current position in June 1998. Most recently, he served as Coordinator of the Interim Secretariat of the World Commission on Dams (1997-1998) and as a Member and Chairman of the Inspection Panel at the World Bank (1994-1997). He worked closely with the Academy during his tenure in senior positions at the U.S. Agency for International Development (1986-1993) as head of the Bureau of Science and

Technology, and as head of the Bureau of Program and Policy Coordination. He has been published widely in the field of political economy, and has taught at Georgetown University as well as the University of Pennsylvania. He received his B.A. from Stanford University (1968) and his M.A. and Ph.D. from Tufts University (1970, 1973).

Deborah Stine is Associate Director of the Committee on Science, Engineering, and Public Policy (COSEPUP). She has worked on various projects throughout the National Academy of Sciences complex since 1989. She received a National Research Council group award for her first study for COSEPUP on policy implications of greenhouse warming, and a Commission on Life Sciences staff citation for her work in risk assessment and management. Other studies have addressed graduate education, responsible conduct of research, careers in science and engineering, environmental remediation, the national biological survey, and corporate environmental stewardship. She holds a bachelor's degree in mechanical and environmental engineering from the University of California, Irvine; a master's degree in business administration; and a PhD in public administration, specializing in policy analysis, from the American University. Before coming to the academy, she was a mathematician for the U.S. Air Force, an air-pollution engineer for the state of Texas, and an air-issues manager for the Chemical Manufacturers Association.

Anne-Marie Mazza is a Senior Program Officer with Committee on Science, Engineering, and Public Policy and the Government-University-Industry Research Roundtable. She staffs COSEPUP on the Research and the Government Performance and Results Act project. She also is responsible for staffing two GUIRR Working Groups: Working Group III, Public Understanding of Science and Technology, chaired by Dr. Ken Shine, and Working Group IV, Human Resources, chaired by Dr. Bruce Alberts. In addition, she serves on the Executive Committee of the Federal

Demonstration Partnership, which GUIRR convenes. She holds a B.A. in Economics, a M.A. in History and Public Policy, and a Ph.D. in Public Policy from The George Washington University. Before coming to the Academy, she was a Senior Consultant at Resource Planning Corporation responsible for a variety of projects involving large-scale litigation, including asbestos, dalkon shield IUD, Times Beach, Love Canal, unintended acceleration in the Audi 5000, and environmental reinsurance.

Brett Willette is the Research Associate for the COSEPUP and Office of Special Projects. He holds a B.S. in Business Management from the University of Maryland and is nearing completion of his M.S. in Healthcare Administration and Policy. Prior to assuming this current position, he served with the U.S. Air Force working on Ballistic Missile Defense Organization weapons systems at the Pentagon from 1995 to 1998 and was Training Development Coordinator for the International Explosive Ordnance Disposal Training School from 1987 to 1995.

Carolyn Ryan holds a bachelors degree in physics from the College of Charleston in Charleston, South Carolina. Just before entering college she lived in Italy for a year as an exchange student. She recently joined the academy as a research associate for COSEPUP and the Office of Special Projects. Previously, she worked with the House of Representatives Committee on Science assisting the Chief Counsel on all issues under the Committee's jurisdiction.

APPENDIX B

HOUSE SCIENCE COMMITTEE LETTER

U.S. HOUSE OF REPRESENTATIVES

COMMITTEE ON SCIENCE

SUITE 2320 RAYBURN HOUSE OFFICE BUILDING
WASHINGTON, DC 20515-6301
(202) 225-6371
TTY: (202) 226-4410
http://www.house.gov/science/welcome.htm

October 23, 1997

Dr. Bruce Alberts
President
National Academy of Sciences
2101 Constitution Avenue, NW
Washington, D.C. 20418

Dear Dr. Alberts:

As you may know, the House Committee on Science is actively involved in the implementation of the Government Performance and Results Act of 1993 (Results Act). The Act requires federal agencies to develop and provide to Congress three basic reports: overseeing five-year strategic plans due this September; annual performance plans to be presented by the Office of Management and Budget next February; and annual performance reports due each year.

The Results Act has the potential to provide information necessary to strengthen program management and improve program performance. This is a challenge for all agencies and in particular those conducting research. At a July 30 hearing before the House Committee on Science, several science-related agencies testified about their efforts to implement the requirements of the Act. It became clear from this hearing that the agencies need to work harder at improving interagency coordination and identifying areas where programs overlap. In the world of research, overlap can be productive and beneficial or it can be duplicative and wasteful -- that is why the agencies must coordinate.

We were pleased to learn of your interest in performing a study to assist with the implementation of the Results Act. We endorse a study that would review how science-related agencies may better incorporate their fundamental research activities into strategic plans and performance plans to improve the management and effectiveness of their science programs. Specifically, we would be interested in a cross-agency comparison of similar types of research.

Of particular interest to us is the development of a thorough interagency coordination process; common outcome-oriented analytic paradigm(s) that could be used across agencies for assessing the results of extramural and intramural fundamental research programs and training and education of the scientific and engineering workforce; and any principles that might assist us in our review of the agencies' performance plans as they relate to research.

Dr. Bruce Alberts
10/23/97
Page 2

Another area for study would be the agencies' implementation of their performance plans, including how they relate to their strategic goals and missions, focusing on the impact of the Results Act on agency programmatic decisions and on the practice of research, the lessons learned from that implementation, and identification of best practices that could be used by other agencies or programs.

In conducting the study, we hope you take the opportunity to hear from the various stakeholders in the process and work with the research agencies. The Committee looks forward to reviewing the results of this effort. If you have any questions please contact Beth Sokul of the Majority Staff (225-0585) or Dan Pearson of the Minority Staff (225-4494).

Sincerely,

F. JAMES SENSENBRENNER, JR.
Chairman
House Committee on Science

GEORGE E. BROWN, JR.
Ranking Democrat
House Committee on Science

PROJECT SUMMARY

The Government Performance and Results Act ("the Results Act") requires all agencies to set goals and to use performance measures for management and budgeting in order to encourage greater efficiency, effectiveness, and accountability in federal programs and spending.

Development of plans to implement the Act has been particularly difficult for agencies responsible for research activities supported by the federal government because of the difficulty of linking results with annual investments in research.

The Committee on Science, Engineering, and Public Policy (COSEPUP) of the National Academy of Sciences, National Academy of Engineering, and Institute of Medicine will conduct a three part study that will seek to

♦ Dialogue with federal agencies, oversight entities, the research community, industry, states, and those in other countries to identify and analyze the most effective approaches to assessing the results of research.

♦ Help the government determine how federal agencies may better incorporate and coordinate their research activities in their strategic plans and performance plans to improve the management and effectiveness of research programs.

> This would include a determination as to what can be reliably measured and the best mechanism for doing so;

what cannot be measured; an evaluation of the extent to which a common analytic paradigm(s) could be used across agencies for assessing the results of extramural and intramural research programs and training and education of the scientific and engineering workforce; development of such a paradigm if feasible; and development of implementation principles and guidelines that could assist Congress and OMB in their review of agency's performance plans.

- Work to develop mechanisms to evaluate the actual impact of implementation of the Act on agency programmatic decisions and on the practices of research, identify lessons learned from implementation, identify best practices that could be used by other agencies or programs, and determine the most effective way for Congress and OMB to use the results of these plans. It will test out those mechanisms to the extent feasible during this timeframe.

GOVERNMENT PERFORMANCE AND RESULTS ACT

S.20

One Hundred Third Congress
of the
United States of America
AT THE FIRST SESSION

Begun and held at the City of Washington on Tuesday, the fifth day of January, one thousand nine hundred and ninety-three

An Act

To provide for the establishment of strategic planning and performance measurement in the Federal Government, and for other purposes.

Be it enacted by the Senate and House of Representatives of the United States of America in Congress assembled,

SECTION 1. SHORT TITLE.

This Act may be cited as the "Government Performance and Results Act of 1993."

SEC. 2. FINDINGS AND PURPOSES.

(a) FINDINGS The Congress finds that—

(1) waste and inefficiency in Federal programs undermine the confidence of the American people in the Government

and reduces the Federal Government's ability to address adequately vital public needs;

(2) Federal managers are seriously disadvantaged in their efforts to improve program efficiency and effectiveness, because of insufficient articulation of program goals and inadequate information on program performance; and

(3) congressional policymaking, spending decisions and program oversight are seriously handicapped by insufficient attention to program performance and results.

(b) PURPOSES The purposes of this Act are to—

(1) improve the confidence of the American people in the capability of the Federal Government, by systematically holding Federal agencies accountable for achieving program results;

(2) initiate program performance reform with a series of pilot projects in setting program goals, measuring program performance against those goals, and reporting publicly on their progress;

(3) improve Federal program effectiveness and public accountability by promoting a new focus on results, service quality, and customer satisfaction;

(4) help Federal managers improve service delivery, by requiring that they plan for meeting program objectives and by providing them with information about program results and service quality;

(5) improve congressional decisionmaking by providing more objective information on achieving statutory objectives, and on the relative effectiveness and efficiency of Federal programs and spending; and

(6) improve internal management of the Federal Government.

SEC. 3. STRATEGIC PLANNING.

Chapter 3 of title 5, United States Code, is amended by adding after section 305 the following new section:

Sec. 306. Strategic plans

(a) No later than September 30, 1997, the head of each agency shall submit to the Director of the Office of Management and Budget and to the Congress a strategic plan for program activities. Such plan shall contain—

(1) a comprehensive mission statement covering the major functions and operations of the agency;

(2) general goals and objectives, including outcome-related goals and objectives, for the major functions and operations of the agency;

(3) a description of how the goals and objectives are to be achieved, including a description of the operational processes, skills and technology, and the human, capital, information, and other resources required to meet those goals and objectives;

(4) a description of how the performance goals included in the plan required by section 1115(a) of title 31 shall be related to the general goals and objectives in the strategic plan;

(5) an identification of those key factors external to the agency and beyond its control that could significantly affect the achievement of the general goals and objectives; and

(6) a description of the program evaluations used in establishing or revising general goals and objectives, with a schedule for future program evaluations.

(b) The strategic plan shall cover a period of not less than five years forward from the fiscal year in which it is submitted, and shall be updated and revised at least every three years.

(c) The performance plan required by section 1115 of title 31 shall be consistent with the agency's strategic plan. A performance plan may not be submitted for a fiscal year not covered by a current strategic plan under this section.

(d) When developing a strategic plan, the agency shall consult with the Congress, and shall solicit and consider the views and suggestions of those entities potentially affected by or interested in such a plan.

(e) The functions and activities of this section shall be considered to be inherently Governmental functions. The drafting of strategic plans under this section shall be performed only by Federal employees.

(f) For purposes of this section the term 'agency' means an Executive agency defined under section 105, but does not include the Central Intelligence Agency, the General Accounting Office, the Panama Canal Commission, the United States Postal Service, and the Postal Rate Commission.

SEC. 4. ANNUAL PERFORMANCE PLANS AND REPORTS.

(a) BUDGET CONTENTS AND SUBMISSION TO CONGRESS Section 1105(a) of title 31, United States Code, is amended by adding at the end thereof the following new paragraph:

> (29) beginning with fiscal year 1999, a Federal Government performance plan for the overall budget as provided for under section 1115.

(b) PERFORMANCE PLANS AND REPORTS Chapter 11 of title 31, United States Code, is amended by adding after section 1114 the following new sections:

Sec. 1115. Performance plans

(a) In carrying out the provisions of section 1105(a)(29), the Director of the Office of Management and Budget shall require each agency to prepare an annual performance plan covering each program activity set forth in the budget of such agency. Such plan shall—

(1) establish performance goals to define the level of performance to be achieved by a program activity;

(2) express such goals in an objective, quantifiable, and measurable form unless authorized to be in an alternative form under subsection (b);

(3) briefly describe the operational processes, skills and technology, and the human, capital, information, or other resources required to meet the performance goals;

(4) establish performance indicators to be used in measuring or assessing the relevant outputs, service levels, and outcomes of each program activity;

(5) provide a basis for comparing actual program results with the established performance goals; and

(6) describe the means to be used to verify and validate measured values.

(b) If an agency, in consultation with the Director of the Office of Management and Budget, determines that it is not feasible to express the performance goals for a particular program activity in an objective, quantifiable, and measurable form, the Director of the Office of Management and Budget may authorize an alternative form. Such alternative form shall—

(1) include separate descriptive statements of—

(A)(i) a minimally effective program, and

(ii) a successful program, or

(B) such alternative as authorized by the Director of the Office of Management and Budget, with sufficient precision and in such terms that would allow for an accurate, independent determination of whether the program activity's performance meets the criteria of the description; or

(2) state why it is infeasible or impractical to express a performance goal in any form for the program activity.

(c) For the purpose of complying with this section, an agency may aggregate, disaggregate, or consolidate program activities, except that any aggregation or consolidation may not omit or minimize the significance of any program activity constituting a major function or operation for the agency.

(d) An agency may submit with its annual performance plan an appendix covering any portion of the plan that—

(1) is specifically authorized under criteria established by an Executive order to be kept secret in the interest of national defense or foreign policy; and

(2) is properly classified pursuant to such Executive order.

(e) The functions and activities of this section shall be considered to be inherently Governmental functions. The drafting of performance plans under this section shall be performed only by Federal employees.

(f) For purposes of this section and sections 1116 through 1119, and sections 9703 and 9704 the term—

(1) "agency" has the same meaning as such term is defined under section 306(f) of title 5;

(2) "outcome measure" means an assessment of the results of a program activity compared to its intended purpose;

(3) "output measure" means the tabulation, calculation, or recording of activity or effort and can be expressed in a quantitative or qualitative manner;

(4) "performance goal" means a target level of performance expressed as a tangible, measurable objective, against which actual achievement can be compared, including a goal expressed as a quantitative standard, value, or rate;

(5) "performance indicator" means a particular value or characteristic used to measure output or outcome;

(6) "program activity" means a specific activity or project as listed in the program and financing schedules of the annual budget of the United States Government; and

(7) "program evaluation" means an assessment, through objective measurement and systematic analysis, of the manner and extent to which Federal programs achieve intended objectives.

Sec. 1116. Program performance reports

(a) No later than March 31, 2000, and no later than March 31 of each year thereafter, the head of each agency shall prepare and submit to the President and the Congress, a report on program performance for the previous fiscal year.

(b)(1) Each program performance report shall set forth the performance indicators established in the agency performance plan under section 1115, along with the actual program performance achieved compared with the performance goals expressed in the plan for that fiscal year.

(2) If performance goals are specified in an alternative form under section 1115(b), the results of such program shall be

described in relation to such specifications, including whether the performance failed to meet the criteria of a minimally effective or successful program.

(c) The report for fiscal year 2000 shall include actual results for the preceding fiscal year, the report for fiscal year 2001 shall include actual results for the two preceding fiscal years, and the report for fiscal year 2002 and all subsequent reports shall include actual results for the three preceding fiscal years.

(d) Each report shall—

(1) review the success of achieving the performance goals of the fiscal year;

(2) evaluate the performance plan for the current fiscal year relative to the performance achieved toward the performance goals in the fiscal year covered by the report;

(3) explain and describe, where a performance goal has not been met (including when a program activity's performance is determined not to have met the criteria of a successful program activity under section 1115(b)(1)(A)(ii) or a corresponding level of achievement if another alternative form is used)—

(A) why the goal was not met;

(B) those plans and schedules for achieving the established performance goal; and

(C) if the performance goal is impractical or infeasible, why that is the case and what action is recommended;

(4) describe the use and assess the effectiveness in achieving performance goals of any waiver under section 9703 of this title; and

(5) include the summary findings of those program evaluations completed during the fiscal year covered by the report.

(e) An agency head may include all program performance information required annually under this section in an annual financial statement required under section 3515 if any such statement is submitted to the Congress no later than March 31 of the applicable fiscal year.

(f) The functions and activities of this section shall be considered to be inherently Governmental functions. The drafting of program performance reports under this section shall be performed only by Federal employees.

Sec. 1117. Exemption

The Director of the Office of Management and Budget may exempt from the requirements of sections 1115 and 1116 of this title and section 306 of title 5, any agency with annual outlays of $20,000,000 or less.

SEC. 5. MANAGERIAL ACCOUNTABILITY AND FLEXIBILITY.

(a) MANAGERIAL ACCOUNTABILITY AND FLEXIBILITY Chapter 97 of title 31, United States Code, is amended by adding after section 9702, the following new section:

Sec. 9703. Managerial accountability and flexibility

(a) Beginning with fiscal year 1999, the performance plans required under section 1115 may include proposals to waive administrative procedural requirements and controls, including specification of personnel staffing levels, limitations on compensation or remuneration, and prohibitions or restrictions on funding transfers among budget object classification 20 and subclassifications 11, 12, 31, and 32 of each annual budget submitted under section 1105, in return for specific individual or organization accountability to achieve a performance goal. In preparing and submitting the performance plan under section 1105(a)(29), the Director of the Office of Management and Budget shall review and may approve any proposed waivers. A waiver shall take effect at the beginning of the fiscal year for which the waiver is approved.

(b) Any such proposal under subsection (a) shall describe the anticipated effects on performance resulting from greater managerial or organizational flexibility, discretion, and authority, and shall quantify the expected improvements in performance resulting from any waiver. The expected improvements shall be compared to current actual performance, and to the projected level of performance that would be achieved independent of any waiver.

(c) Any proposal waiving limitations on compensation or remuneration shall precisely express the monetary change in compensation or remuneration amounts, such as bonuses or awards, that shall result from meeting, exceeding, or failing to meet performance goals.

(d) Any proposed waiver of procedural requirements or controls imposed by an agency (other than the proposing agency or the Office of Management and Budget) may not be included in a performance plan unless it is endorsed by the agency that established the requirement, and the endorsement included in the proposing agency's performance plan.

(e) A waiver shall be in effect for one or two years as specified by the Director of the Office of Management and Budget in approving the waiver. A waiver may be renewed for a subsequent year. After a waiver has been in effect for three consecutive years, the performance plan prepared under section 1115 may propose that a waiver, other than a waiver of limitations on compensation or remuneration, be made permanent.

(f) For purposes of this section, the definitions under section 1115(f) shall apply.

SEC. 6. PILOT PROJECTS.

(a) PERFORMANCE PLANS AND REPORTS Chapter 11 of title 31, United States Code, is amended by inserting after section 1117 (as added by section 4 of this Act) the following new section:

Sec. 1118. Pilot projects for performance goals

(a) The Director of the Office of Management and Budget, after consultation with the head of each agency, shall designate not less than ten agencies as pilot projects in performance measurement for fiscal years 1994, 1995, and 1996. The selected agencies shall reflect a representative range of Government functions and capabilities in measuring and reporting program performance.

(b) Pilot projects in the designated agencies shall undertake the preparation of performance plans under section 1115, and program performance reports under section 1116, other than section 1116(c), for one or more of the major functions and operations of the agency. A strategic plan shall be used when preparing agency performance plans during one or more years of the pilot period.

(c) No later than May 1, 1997, the Director of the Office of Management and Budget shall submit a report to the President and to the Congress which shall—

(1) assess the benefits, costs, and usefulness of the plans and reports prepared by the pilot agencies in meeting the

purposes of the Government Performance and Results Act of 1993;

(2) identify any significant difficulties experienced by the pilot agencies in preparing plans and reports; and

(3) set forth any recommended changes in the requirements of the provisions of Government Performance and Results Act of 1993, section 306 of title 5, sections 1105, 1115, 1116, 1117, 1119 and 9703 of this title, and this section.

(b) MANAGERIAL ACCOUNTABILITY AND FLEXIBILITY Chapter 97 of title 31, United States Code, is amended by inserting after section 9703 (as added by section 5 of a representative range of Government functions and capabilities in measuring and reporting program performance.

Sec. 9704. Pilot projects for managerial accountability and flexibility

(a) The Director of the Office of Management and Budget shall designate not less than five agencies as pilot projects in managerial accountability and flexibility for fiscal years 1995 and 1996. Such agencies shall be selected from those designated as pilot projects under section 1118 and shall reflect a representative range of Government functions and capabilities in measuring and reporting program performance.

(b) Pilot projects in the designated agencies shall include proposed waivers in accordance with section 9703 for one or more of the major functions and operations of the agency.

(c) The Director of the Office of Management and Budget shall include in the report to the President and to the Congress required under section 1118(c)—

(1) an assessment of the benefits, costs, and usefulness of

increasing managerial and organizational flexibility, discretion, and authority in exchange for improved performance through a waiver; and

(2) an identification of any significant difficulties experienced by the pilot agencies in preparing proposed waivers.

(d) For purposes of this section the definitions under section 1115(f) shall apply.

(c) PERFORMANCE BUDGETING Chapter 11 of title 31, United States Code, is amended by inserting after section 1118 (as added by section 6 of this Act) the following new section:

Sec. 1119. Pilot projects for performance budgeting

(a) The Director of the Office of Management and Budget, after consultation with the head of each agency shall designate not less than five agencies as pilot projects in performance budgeting for fiscal years 1998 and 1999. At least three of the agencies shall be selected from those designated as pilot projects under section 1118, and shall also reflect a representative range of Government functions and capabilities in measuring and reporting program performance.

(b) Pilot projects in the designated agencies shall cover the preparation of performance budgets. Such budgets shall present, for one or more of the major functions and operations of the agency, the varying levels of performance, including outcome-related performance, that would result from different budgeted amounts.

(c) The Director of the Office of Management and Budget shall include, as an alternative budget presentation in the budget submitted under section 1105 for fiscal year 1999, the performance budgets of the designated agencies for this fiscal year.

(d) No later than March 31, 2001, the Director of the Office of

Management and Budget shall transmit a report to the President and to the Congress on the performance budgeting pilot projects which shall—

(1) assess the feasibility and advisability of including a performance budget as part of the annual budget submitted under section 1105;

(2) describe any difficulties encountered by the pilot agencies in preparing a performance budget;

(3) recommend whether legislation requiring performance budgets should be proposed and the general provisions of any legislation; and

(4) set forth any recommended changes in the other requirements of the Government Performance and Results Act of 1993, section 306 of title 5, sections 1105, 1115, 1116, 1117, and 9703 of this title, and this section.

(e) After receipt of the report required under subsection (d), the Congress may specify that a performance budget be submitted as part of the annual budget submitted under section 1105.

SEC. 7. UNITED STATES POSTAL SERVICE.

Part III of title 39, United States Code, is amended by adding at the end thereof the following new chapter:

CHAPTER 28—STRATEGIC PLANNING AND PERFORMANCE MANAGEMENT

Sec.

2801. Definitions.
2802. Strategic plans.
2803. Performance plans.
2804. Program performance reports.

2805. Inherently Governmental functions.

Sec. 2801. Definitions

For purposes of this chapter the term—

(1) "outcome measure" refers to an assessment of the results of a program activity compared to its intended purpose;

(2) "output measure" refers to the tabulation, calculation, or recording of activity or effort and can be expressed in a quantitative or qualitative manner;

(3) "performance goal" means a target level of performance expressed as a tangible, measurable objective, against which actual achievement shall be compared, including a goal expressed as a quantitative standard, value, or rate;

(4) "performance indicator" refers to a particular value or characteristic used to measure output or outcome;

(5) "program activity" means a specific activity related to the mission of the Postal Service; and

(6) "program evaluation" means an assessment, through objective measurement and systematic analysis, of the manner and extent to which Postal Service programs achieve intended objectives.

Sec. 2802. Strategic plans

(a) No later than September 30, 1997, the Postal Service shall submit to the President and the Congress a strategic plan for its program activities. Such plan shall contain—

(1) a comprehensive mission statement covering the major functions and operations of the Postal Service;

(2) general goals and objectives, including outcome-related goals and objectives, for the major functions and operations

of the Postal Service;

(3) a description of how the goals and objectives are to be achieved, including a description of the operational processes, skills and technology, and the human, capital, information, and other resources required to meet those goals and objectives;

(4) a description of how the performance goals included in the plan required under section 2803 shall be related to the general goals and objectives in the strategic plan;

(5) an identification of those key factors external to the Postal Service and beyond its control that could significantly affect the achievement of the general goals and objectives; and

(6) a description of the program evaluations used in establishing or revising general goals and objectives, with a schedule for future program evaluations.

(b) The strategic plan shall cover a period of not less than five years forward from the fiscal year in which it is submitted, and shall be updated and revised at least every three years.

(c) The performance plan required under section 2803 shall be consistent with the Postal Service's strategic plan. A performance plan may not be submitted for a fiscal year not covered by a current strategic plan under this section.

(d) When developing a strategic plan, the Postal Service shall solicit and consider the views and suggestions of those entities potentially affected by or interested in such a plan, and shall advise the Congress of the contents of the plan.

Sec. 2803. Performance plans

(a) The Postal Service shall prepare an annual performance

plan covering each program activity set forth in the Postal Service budget, which shall be included in the comprehensive statement presented under section 2401(g) of this title. Such plan shall—

(1) establish performance goals to define the level of performance to be achieved by a program activity;

(2) express such goals in an objective, quantifiable, and measurable form unless an alternative form is used under subsection (b);

(3) briefly describe the operational processes, skills and technology, and the human, capital, information, or other resources required to meet the performance goals;

(4) establish performance indicators to be used in measuring or assessing the relevant outputs, service levels, and outcomes of each program activity;

(5) provide a basis for comparing actual program results with the established performance goals; and

(6) describe the means to be used to verify and validate measured values.

(b) If the Postal Service determines that it is not feasible to express the performance goals for a particular program activity in an objective, quantifiable, and measurable form, the Postal Service may use an alternative form. Such alternative form shall—

(1) include separate descriptive statements of—

(A) a minimally effective program, and

(B) a successful program,

with sufficient precision and in such terms that would allow for an accurate, independent determination of whether the program activity's performance meets the criteria of either description; or

(2) state why it is infeasible or impractical to express a performance goal in any form for the program activity.

(c) In preparing a comprehensive and informative plan under this section, the Postal Service may aggregate, disaggregate, or consolidate program activities, except that any aggregation or consolidation may not omit or minimize the significance of any program activity constituting a major function or operation.

(d) The Postal Service may prepare a non-public annex to its plan covering program activities or parts of program activities relating to—

(1) the avoidance of interference with criminal prosecution; or

(2) matters otherwise exempt from public disclosure under section 410(c) of this title.

Sec. 2804. Program performance reports

(a) The Postal Service shall prepare a report on program performance for each fiscal year, which shall be included in the annual comprehensive statement presented under section 2401(g) of this title.

(b)(1) The program performance report shall set forth the performance indicators established in the Postal Service performance plan, along with the actual program performance achieved compared with the performance goals expressed in the plan for that fiscal year.

(2) If performance goals are specified by descriptive statements of a minimally effective program activity and a successful program activity, the results of such program shall be described

in relationship to those categories, including whether the performance failed to meet the criteria of either category.

(c) The report for fiscal year 2000 shall include actual results for the preceding fiscal year, the report for fiscal year 2001 shall include actual results for the two preceding fiscal years, and the report for fiscal year 2002 and all subsequent reports shall include actual results for the three preceding fiscal years.

(d) Each report shall—

(1) review the success of achieving the performance goals of the fiscal year;

(2) evaluate the performance plan for the current fiscal year relative to the performance achieved towards the performance goals in the fiscal year covered by the report;

(3) explain and describe, where a performance goal has not been met (including when a program activity's performance is determined not to have met the criteria of a successful program activity under section 2803(b)(2))—

(A) why the goal was not met;

(B) those plans and schedules for achieving the established performance goal; and

(C) if the performance goal is impractical or infeasible, why that is the case and what action is recommended; and

(4) include the summary findings of those program evaluations completed during the fiscal year covered by the report.

Sec. 2805. Inherently Governmental functions

The functions and activities of this chapter shall be considered to be inherently Governmental functions. The drafting of strategic plans, performance plans, and program performance reports under this section shall be performed only by employees of the Postal Service.

SEC. 8. CONGRESSIONAL OVERSIGHT AND LEGISLATION.

(a) IN GENERAL Nothing in this Act shall be construed as limiting the ability of Congress to establish, amend, suspend, or annul a performance goal. Any such action shall have the effect of superseding that goal in the plan submitted under section 1105(a)(29) of title 31, United States Code.

(b) GAO REPORT No later than June 1, 1997, the Comptroller General of the United States shall report to Congress on the implementation of this Act, including the prospects for compliance by Federal agencies beyond those participating as pilot projects under sections 1118 and 9704 of title 31, United States Code.

SEC. 9. TRAINING.

The Office of Personnel Management shall, in consultation with the Director of the Office of Management and Budget and the Comptroller General of the United States, develop a strategic planning and performance measurement training component for its management training program and otherwise provide managers with an orientation on the development and use of strategic planning and program performance measurement.

SEC. 10. APPLICATION OF ACT.

No provision or amendment made by this Act may be construed as—

(1) creating any right, privilege, benefit, or entitlement for any person who is not an officer or employee of the United States acting in such capacity, and no person who is not an

officer or employee of the United States acting in such capacity shall have standing to file any civil action in a court of the United States to enforce any provision or amendment made by this Act; or

(2) superseding any statutory requirement, including any requirement under section 553 of title 5, United States Code.

SEC. 11. TECHNICAL AND CONFORMING AMENDMENTS.

(a) AMENDMENT TO TITLE 5, UNITED STATES CODE The table of sections for chapter 3 of title 5, United States Code, is amended by adding after the item relating to section 305 the following:

306. Strategic plans.

(b) AMENDMENTS TO TITLE 31, UNITED STATES CODE

(1) AMENDMENT TO CHAPTER 11 The table of sections for chapter 11 of title 31, United States Code, is amended by adding after the item relating to section 1114 the following:

1115. Performance plans.

1116. Program performance reports.

1117. Exemptions.

1118. Pilot projects for performance goals.

1119. Pilot projects for performance budgeting.

(2) AMENDMENT TO CHAPTER 97 The table of sections for chapter 97 of title 31, United States Code, is amended by adding after the item relating to section 9702 the following:

9703. Managerial accountability and flexibility.

9704. Pilot projects for managerial accountability and flexibility.

(c) AMENDMENT TO TITLE 39, UNITED STATES CODE The table of chapters for part III of title 39, United States Code, is amended by adding at the end thereof the following new item:

2801.

Speaker of the House of Representatives.

Vice President of the United States and

President of the Senate.

REFERENCES

American Enterprise Institute, Brookings Institution, and National Science Foundation Directorate for Social and Behavior Sciences, "Conference on the Contributions of Research to the Economy and Society," (Washington, D.C. October 3, 1994).

Anderson, Richard C., F. Narin, Paul McAllister "Publication Ratings versus Peer Ratings of Universities" Journal of the American Society for Information Science March (1978) 91-103.

Atkinson, Richard C. and William A. Blanpied, Peer Review and the Public Interest, Issues in Science and Technology, vol 1. no. 4, 1985.

Bozeman, B. and J. Melkers, "Peer Review and Evaluation of R&D Impacts," Evaluating R&D Impacts, Kluwer Academic Publishers, Norwell, Mass., (1993) 79-98.

Carnegie Commission on Science, Technology, and Government. Enabling the Future: Linking Science and Technology to Societal Goals (Carnegie Commission: New York, NY 1992).

Cole, J. and S. Cole, Peer Review in the National Science Foundation, Washington, D.C.: National Academy Press, 1981.

Commission on Physical Sciences, Mathematics, and Applications, (1995) Research Restructuring and Assessment, National Academy Press, Washington, D.C.

Committee on Science, Engineering, and Public Policy, (1982) The Quality of Research in Science, National Academy Press, Washington, D.C.

Committee on Science, Engineering, and Public Policy, (1993) Science, Technology, and the Federal Government: National Goals for a New Era, National Academy Press, Washington, D.C.

Committee on Science, Engineering, and Public Policy, (1997) International Benchmarking of U.S. Mathematics, National Academy Press, Washington, D.C.

Committee on Science, Engineering, and Public Policy, (1998) International Benchmarking of U.S. Material Sciences and Engineering Research, National Academy Press, Washington, D.C.

Landau, Ralph, Technology, Economics, and Public Policy. In Landau, Ralph and Dale W. Jorgensen, eds. Technology and Economic Policy. Cambridge, Ballinger Publ. Co., 1986.

Nadiri, M. Ishaq. "Innovations and Technological Spillovers," Working Paper No. 4423 (National Bureau of Economic Research: Cambridge, MA, August 1993).

National Academy of Sciences, 1996, Beyond Discovery: The Path from Research to Human Benefit, The Global Positioning System: The Role of Atomic Clocks, http://www2.nas.edu/bsi/2132.html.

National Science and Technology Council, (1996) Assessing Fundamental Science, Washington, D.C.

Small, Henry G. "A Co-Citation Model of a Scientific Specialty: A Longitudinal Study of Collagen Research" Social Studies of Science Vol. 7 (1977), 139-66.

U.S. Government Accounting Office, Peer Review; Reforms Needed to Ensure Fairness in Federal Agency Grant Selection, June 1984.

U.S. General Accounting Office, (1997) The Government Performance and Results Act: 1997 Governmentwide Implementation Will Be Uneven,Washington, D.C.

Agency Strategic and Performance Plans Web Locations

Government Wide Performance Plan:

http://www.whitehouse.gov/WH/EOP/OMB/html/gpptoc.htm

General Accounting Office

http://www.gao.gov/special.pubs/publist.htm

General Pages of Some Agencies:

http://www.ombwatch.org/www/ombw/gpra/gprasp.html

http://www.govexec.com/dailyfed/0997/090897b1.htm

http://server.conginst.org/conginst/results/index.html

Department of Agriculture

Strategic Plan: http://www.usda.gov/ocfo/strat/

Performance Plan: http://www.usda.gov/ocfo/annlplan/index.html

Department of Defense

Strategic Plan: http://www.defenselink.mil/pubs/qdr/

Performance Plan: http://www.dtic.mil/execsec/adr98/apdx_j.html

Department of Energy

Strategic Plan: http://www.doe.gov/policy/doeplan.html

Performance Plan: http:// www.doe.gov/policy/sol98/index.htm

Department of Health and Human Services

Strategic Plan: http://aspe.os.dhhs.gov/hhsplan/intro.htm

Performance Plan: http://www.hhs.gov/progorg/asmb/budget/fy99budget

Department of Transportation

Strategic Plan: http://www.dot.gov/hot/dotplan.html

Performance Plan: http://ostpxweb.dot.gov/budget/perfp99.htm

Environmental Protection Agency

Strategic Plan: http://www.epa.gov/ocfopage/plantoc.htm

Performance Plan: http://www.epa.gov/ocfo/99budget/1999bib.htm

National Aeronautics and Space Administration

Strategic Plan: http://www.hq.nasa.gov/office/nsp/

National Oceanic and Atmospheric Administration

Strategic Plan: http://www.noaa.gov/str-plan/

Performance Plan: http://www.doc.gov/bmi/budget/strtgc/strtone.htm

National Institute of Standards and Technology

Strategic Plan: http://www.doc.gov/bmi

Performance Plan: http://www.doc.gov/bmi/budget/strtgc/strtone.htm

National Science Foundation

Strategic Plan: http://www.nsf.gov/od/gpraplan/gpraplan.htm

Performance Plan: http://www.nsf.gov/pubs/1998/nsf99gprapp/start.htm